Vegan Diet

For Beginners

The Ultimate Beginner's Vegan Diet Guide & Cookbook – Easy To Do Cookbook Recipes to Lose Weight and Stay Healthy + 30 Delicious Recipes

By Simone Jacobs

For more great books visit:

HMWPublishing.com

Get another book for Free

I want to thank you for purchasing this book and offer you another book (just as long and valuable as this book), "Health & Fitness Mistakes You Don't Know You're Making", completely free.

Visit the link below to signup and receive it:

www.hmwpublishing.com/gift

In this book, I will break down the most common health & fitness mistakes, you are probably committing right now, and I will reveal how you can easily get in the best shape of your life!

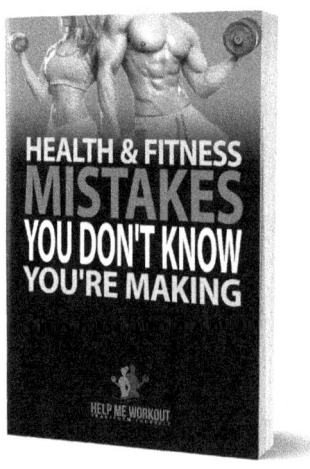

In addition to this valuable gift, you will also have an opportunity to get our new books for free, enter giveaways, and receive other valuable emails from me. Again, visit the link to sign up:

www.hmwpublishing.com/gift

TABLE OF CONTENTS

Introduction 9

Chapter 1: The Basics of Going Vegan 11

    Different Types of Vegan Diets 12

    Before You Make the Big Move 15

    What Truly is a Vegan Diet 22

    Getting the Vegan Myths Out of the Way 23

Chapter 2: The Health Benefits of a Vegan Diet 27

    Is It the Right Decision for You? 27

    Health 28

    Environment 29

    Ethical 30

    Going Vegan and Losing Weight 31

    Understanding Vegan Nutrition 32

Fat 32

Omega 3 Fatty Acids......................33

Protein 33

Vitamin D and Vitamin B12 35

Calcium 35

Other Minerals...................................36

Chapter 3: How to Transition to a Vegan Diet..38

Transitioning Into Plant-based Foods 38

Equipping Your Kitchen the Right Way...42

Sticking to a Brand New Lifestyle 45

Chapter 4: Avoiding These Common Mistakes 49

Avoiding the Risks of Veganism...............49

Writing Your Vegan Diet Plan 53

Nutritional Features of Your Vegan Diet .56

Caloric Macros (Macronutrients).............56

Chapter 5: Vegan Breakfast Recipes .62

Chive Waffles with Soy Mushrooms and Maple 62

Avocado Salsa and Mexican Beans on Toast 66

Lemon Poppy Scones 68

Vegan Crepes 70

Garbanzo-Oat Pancakes 72

Chapter 6: Vegan Lunch Recipes 74

Seitan and Black Bean Stir-fry 74

Eggless Tofu Spinach Quiche 77

Vegan Mac and No Cheese 79

Tomato, Basil, and Olive Oil Pasta...........81

Carrot Rice Nut Burger.............................83

Chapter 7: Vegan Dinner Recipes......85

Sweet Potato and Coconut Curry 85

Vegan Shepherd's Pie 89

Roast Summer Vegetables and Chickpeas 92

Veggies and Tofu in Peanut Sauce 94

Vegan Fajitas 96

Chapter 8: Vegan Dessert Recipes 98

Vegan Carrot Cake 98

Salted Caramel Biscuit Bar 102

Mint-Chip Coconut Milk Ice Cream 105

Orange Vegan Cake 107

Vegan Rose Meringues 109

Chapter 9: Vegan Soups, Stews and Salads 111

Crunchy Bulgur Salad..............................111

Tomato Soup...114

Barley and Lentil Stew............................117

Spinach and Lentil Soup 119

Black Bean and Corn Salad 121

Chapter 10: Vegan Snack and Smoothie Recipe 123

Strawberry and Oatmeal Smoothie 123

Sweet Potato, Chili, and Peanut Butter Quesadillas...125

Raw Strawberry Jam 128

Vegan Cashew Cream Cheese 130

Kale and Banana Smoothie 132

Bonus Chapter: 14-Day Vegan Getting Started Plan......................................133

Final Words..138

Introduction

I want to thank you and congratulate you for purchasing the *"Vegan Diet for Beginners: The Ultimate Beginner's Vegan Guide & Cookbook."*

This book takes you on a spectacular journey with food and vegetables, specifically. If you do not already have a love affair with your friendly veggies, it is about time that you learn how to take advantage of the many benefits it offers. Veganism is not a fad it is a lifestyle—and you are getting the best guide through the whole journey, with this book. Thanks again for purchasing this book, I hope you enjoy reading it!

Also, before you get started, I recommend you joining our email newsletter to receive updates on any upcoming new book releases or promotions. You can sign-up for free, and as a bonus, you will receive a free gift. Our *"Health & Fitness Mistakes You Don't Know You're Making"* book! This book has been written to demystify, expose the top do's and don'ts and to finally equip you with the information you need to get in the best shape of your life. Due to the overwhelming amount of misinformation and lies told by magazines and self-proclaimed "gurus", it's becoming harder and harder to get reliable information to get in shape. As opposed to having to go through dozens of biased, unreliable and un-trustworthy sources to get your health & fitness information. Everything you need to help you has been broken down in this book for you to easily follow and to immediately get results to achieve your desired fitness goals in the shortest amount of time.

Once again, to join our free email newsletter and to receive a free copy of this valuable book, please visit the link and signup now: www.hmwpublishing.com/gift

Chapter 1: The Basics of Going Vegan

Veganism is a specific diet that involves complete abstinence from all kinds of animal products. And those who decide to become vegan, do so because of the following reason:

1. Dietary Veganism. It is strict veganism, and when you follow this type of diet, you stay away from all kinds of animal products including dairy products and eggs. Anything that is an animal source should be avoided.

2. Ethical Veganism. It is a type of veganism that goes over and beyond the food restrictions because a person who is an ethical vegan will also abstain from the use of animals and animal products, for any purpose—like clothing.

3. Environmental Veganism. It is a type of veganism borne from the understanding that the means in which animal products are obtained is damaging to the environment.

Are you thinking of going vegan? Are you thinking of making the big leap but you are worried about a lot of things? In the next pages, you will discover enough to gain comfortable footing over the journey you are contemplating taking or gain even greater insights if you have already commited to be a vegan.

Different Types of Vegan Diets

You have looked into the common reasons why people decide to go Vegan. Here is a list of the different types of Vegan Diets. If you are exploring which direction to go, know that you can choose to be either one of these:

1. Ethical Vegan – As mentioned in the previous page, an ethical vegan is someone who abstains from the intake of all kinds of animals and animal by-products such as meat, cheese, honey, dairy, eggs, and fish. Aside from that, they do not wear clothing or accessories made from animals such as silk, leather, and fur; and they do not use cosmetic products tested on animals. Sometimes their moral stand goes over beyond consumption; as they can boycott a store that sells any animal products. Circuses and zoos are a disgrace to them; and their position as a vegan is born from their belief that all living beings are equal, so animals should not be exploited, in any way.

2. Plant Based Vegan – Many plant-based vegans decide to go vegan because of health reasons. Their diet is not very strict, and so they may consume honey or fish oil; and unlike ethical vegans, they may not refrain from the use of animal as clothing and so forth.

3. Raw Vegan – A person who chooses to become a raw vegan to embrace the health benefit it brings. Their diet is strict because apart from abstaining from animals or animal by-products, they do not consume anything that cooked above 115°F. Cooking usually depletes vegetables of their essential nutrients. A raw vegan's diet will be composed of vegetables, fruits, nuts, sprouts, seeds, roots, natural spices, fresh herbs, cold pressed oils, raw nut butters, raw nut milk, seaweeds, unprocessed olives, dried fruits, unpasteurized soy sauce, raw cocoa powder, vinegars, and pure maple syrup.

4. Junk Food Vegan – A junk food vegan is someone who is an ethical vegan, but is not at all concerned about the health benefits of going vegan. It means that they do not embrace the health feature of the diet, and may consume vegan junk food, quite excessively. It is proof that going vegan does not automatically mean that you are eating healthily.

Before You Make the Big Move

In whatever you do, it's nice to get the advice of experts. Especially if you are about to do something for the first time, and you have no clue about it, some tips will be of value.

Before the big move, here are some things you have to know:

1. *Do not be in a hurry.* The journey is not going to be easy, but it will be a fruitful one, especially when you complete it. Regardless of how big the mountain you have ahead of you, though, you should take your own pace. Try not to be in a hurry. Believe that you will get there, one-step-at-a-time. If you have to go one-animal-product-at-a-time, do it that way. If you want to start with one vegan meal a day, go ahead. The point is for you to get there—it doesn't matter how or how fast.

2. *Focus on the fruits and vegetables.* The big mistake people make about going vegan is they have too much of the starch products such as potatoes, pasta, rice, and bread. To compensate for the absence of meats, they fill up on starch which is rich in vitamins and nutrients like vegetables and fruits.

3. Do not be afraid to experiment. A lot of people think that vegans are malnourished, but that is not true. You should be more open about exploring the world of veganism so that you can maximize its full benefits. Play with tastes and open yourself up to new dishes, so that you can broaden your horizon.

4. Choose whole grains. Instead of having a lot of pasta and bread, choose whole grains, instead. They will also be a good source of protein, so make sure to pack on various types of grains.

5. **Find the right support.** People say that you get by with the help of friends and there is value in that, especially when you are a "baby" vegan. Working with a group is good because you become accountable to each other. You have someone to who will nag, remind, motivate, inspire, and guide you through it all. You can share experiences, tips, burdens, and so forth.

6. **Decide about how you acquire the food.** This may seem ridiculous, but it is crucial. Are you going to be cooking the food or are you going to pay for vegan food delivery? You have to realize that making the right food choices is going to be very difficult, so you need to be in complete control. By cooking your food you will know for sure what is on your plate—ordering from a vegan catering serving is good because it takes away the pressure from you, but you hardly have any choice about what gets delivered to your house. Still, these options will be easier compared to scouring a menu in a restaurant to see what fits into your diet.

7. *Declutter your life*. Rid yourself of old habits. Starting from the house, you have to clean your refrigerator and pantry to remove anything that goes against your new diet. Also, you have to make changes to your routine—less convenience store and fast food visits, unless you are sure that it fits in with your new lifestyle.

8. *Study the diet closely*. Eventually, you will get the hang of it, but as a newbie, you may feel completely lost. Before you begin, you have to give yourself some time to learn. This book is an excellent way to start because it will provide you with a rundown of all the stuff you have to know. Do not be content with knowing little. If you are going to do this, you have to do this right, so you need to study it. Your goal is to master the diet, even with your eyes closed. That way you can be confident that things won't go wrong.

9. Be kind to yourself. It will be hard, and you will have slip ups, but one or a few days should not define your journey so do not beat yourself up. If you fall, get back on the ride and keep on going. Do not be quick to abandon your journey—it will be worth it in the end.

10. Learn how to supplement. There are certain things that your diet may be lacking, such as iron, so you need to take supplements. You cannot deprive yourself of what it needs to function efficiently, so you look closely into your diet and determine what supplements you need to add.

What Truly is a Vegan Diet

There is a big question marks looming over the whole vegan phenomenon. People seem to be confused with the terms and inclusions, so if you are going to embark on this for real, you have to be fully aware.

The confusion is between Veganism and Vegetarianism. Vegetarians do not eat poultry, fish, and meat. Vegans are vegetarians who also do not eat or use dairy products, eggs, cosmetics, wool, silk, and soaps manufactured from animal products.

Based on the discussion earlier, one can choose to be vegan for a lot of reasons:

- Health
- Environment
- Ethics

Why do you want to be a vegan? The phenomenon of veganism can be traced back as early as 1944. However, it was in 1949 that Leslie J Cross gave its first definition: "The principle of the emancipation of animals from exploitation by man to seek an end to the use of animals by man for food, commodities, work, vivisection and by all other uses involving exploitation of animal by man."

This definition has evolved since, but, regarding food, a vegan's diet will be consist of vegetables, fruits, seeds, grains, nuts, pulses, and beans.

Getting the Vegan Myths Out of the Way

There are mixed reviews about the vegan diet, and if you are having doubts, it may be that you are concerned about some of the myths. Before you begin, it is necessary that you get these myths out of the way, to avoid the confusion. You have to understand veganism as a whole before you decide about it, so it's time for you to face the truth:

- **"The food is bland and boring."** People think vegan food has no character, but that is completely wrong. This book will give you fantastic 100% vegan recipes that are mouthwatering. There are so many ways to dress a bowl of vegetables if you know what to do. And about missing out on all the food, you are used to, understand that if you know where to look, there are vegan alternatives that will satisfy every craving you have.

- **"You will get frail and weak."** People have this thinking that the vegan diet is insufficient of everything necessary, so you will feel weak because your body is continually lacking. Do you know that many athletes maintain a strict vegan diet? A plant-based diet can sufficiently supply you with what you need, as long as you know how to do it right.

- **"It is not healthy."** In a nutshell, vegan is low-fat, and is a strict plant-based diet and is known to reverse and improve health conditions for people with heart disease and diabetes. It also prevents obesity, which is a rising problem, worldwide. How is that not healthy, at all? Still, vegan does not automatically mean it is healthy, mainly if you consume a lot of the vegan junk food. But ideally, the most simplistic form of this diet is very beneficial for your health.
- **"It is expensive to maintain."** Stick to the staples—bananas, potatoes, grains, and beans, because they are not just the healthiest, they are also the most convenient to have. If you know how to play with these ingredients, you will realize that the vegan diet is very cost-effective. And have you ever checked out how cheap vegetables are? It does not have to be wholefoods—you just have to know how to use the food that you can have.

- "Eating out is going to be a nightmare." People are so afraid to make the change to vegan because they think that eating out will be so difficult. If you know the vegan diet, through and through, you will realize that there are so many options for you. Also, there are more vegan places now, so it will not be so difficult. You can even ask the waiter for a vegan alternative to a dish you wish to order if you want to make things easier for yourself.

- "You will lack in protein." Since you are not eating meat, do you know where to source your protein from? Protein can be obtained from beans, nuts, pulses, and peas. You should not lack in protein if you include enough of these in your diet.

Chapter 2: The Health Benefits of a Vegan Diet

Just because you are taking on the vegan route doesn't mean you are the epitome of health. But the most carefully planned vegan diet can be very beneficial to your health and well-being.

Is It the Right Decision for You?

Why should you go vegan? Of the many diet disciplines around, why should you single out veganism? People choose to be vegan for three main things, their health, the environment, and for ethical reasons.

If you want to solidify your movement, you may want to understand the three aspects intimately:

Regarding health, you make the turn to veganism and embrace the world of fruits and vegetables because you realize that they are your safest bets against all kinds of diseases:

- Cancer (Colon Cancer and Prostate Cancer)
- Cardiovascular Disease
- Hypertension
- Ischemic Heart Disease
- Obesity
- Stroke
- Type 2 Diabetes

The world is very toxic. There are a lot of potential poisons in the food world and when you finally realize the impact of this fact, know that you can make a turn to vegan and change your life. A well-constructed vegan meal plan can be very healthy. Your vegan lifestyle can very well prolong your life and improve the quality of life that you live.

Environment

Food is a necessity. Food production has become a priority, and it has been a big deal for a long time, but the world will be unable to sustain the agricultural impacts if it continues at the current rate. The demand for animal products has significantly risen through the years, so going vegan is also deciding to save the planet.

The practices involved in food production heavily exploit the planet's natural resources. If this goes on, conditions will get worse, and eventually, there would not be enough food to feed everyone.

You should understand that adopting a vegan lifestyle is going to result in less carbon footprint. So it is more than making a healthy choice for your body, you are also making a healthy turn for the planet (and everyone else in it).

Ethical

Have you given any thought to how the chicken on your plate got to your dinner table? The world has long enjoyed the consumption of meat while being oblivious to the awful truth involved in the slaughter of animals for food.

You do not have to be an animal lover to make this stand. But many of the known methods are very invasive, and the only way that you can actively take a move against these unhealthy practices is to refuse to support it. Your turn to veganism says to the world that you are the kind of person who will not sit and pretend it's okay to harm animals.

Those who choose to go vegan make this decision wholeheartedly, be it for their health, the environment, or animal welfare. Knowing what you know now, do you think this is the right decision for you?

Going Vegan and Losing Weight

Obesity is a leading world problem and a lot of lives are lost, every day, due to the ill-effects of obesity. Somehow, everything spirals down when you begin packing on extra pounds. Although being fit does not guarantee optimum health, obesity is not something you should be okay with.

Veganism and weight loss are mostly dependent on the high fiber content of vegetables and fruits. Fiber, if you do not know, is like a vacuum in your system. When you have a lot of fiber, your body will be more efficient at cleaning your digestive tract of toxins. Apart from its cleansing properties, vegetables are extremely low in calories so that it will help in weight control compared to another kind of diet.

Understanding Vegan Nutrition

So how can you maximize the full benefits of going vegan? It all sounds good on paper but how can you apply this lifestyle so that your body receives the right amount of nutrition it needs?

Fat

While you think you are being smart about missing out on the fat, by going vegan, the body still needs to be supplied with fat. To support this, you can source your fat from the following:

- Avocado

- Coconut
- Nut butter (cashew butter, peanut butter, walnut butter, almond butter, hazelnut butter)
- Nuts
- Oils (coconut oils, olive oil, avocado oil, canola oil, rice bran oil)
- Seed butter (pumpkin seed butter, sunflower butter, hemp seed butter)

Omega 3 Fatty Acids

A healthy kind of fat, you can get omega-3 fatty acids from canola oil, flaxseed, flaxseed oil, soybeans, tofu, and walnuts.

Protein

People think that protein is only sourced from animals and animal by-products. The body needs it because muscles and bones rely on it for healthy structure and repair. If you are going vegan, you will obtain your protein from:

- Almonds
- Broccoli
- Chickpeas
- Kale
- Lentils
- Peanut butter
- Peas
- Potatoes
- Rice
- Soy milk
- Spinach
- Tofu
- Whole wheat bread

Vitamin D and Vitamin B12

Vitamin D is not easily obtained in the vegan diet. B12, on the other hand, is scarce, but the demand is quite low. Regardless, you need to supply your diet accordingly. Of course, the most natural source of Vitamin D is still sunshine, but you can also obtain it from Vitamin D-fortified rice milk and soy milk. In the case of Vitamin B12, its vegan sources are:

- Red star nutritional yeast (vegetarian sports formula)
- Miso
- Seaweed
- Tempeh

Calcium

There is no doubt that the body needs calcium, zinc, iron and all kinds of minerals. Calcium is necessary for healthy bones, and they are obtained from the following sources:

- Almonds

- Blackstrap molasses
- Calcium-fortified soy milk
- Calcium-fortified orange juice
- Dark green vegetables
- Soybeans
- Soy yogurt
- Tahini
- Tofu

Other Minerals

Iron, which is necessary for blood health, is conveniently sourced from the following:

- Beet greens
- Black beans
- Black-eyed peas
- Blackstrap molasses
- Bokchoi
- Bulghur
- Chickpeas
- Kale
- Kidney beans

- Lentils
- Peas
- Prune juice
- Raisins
- Soybeans
- Swiss chard
- Tahini
- Tempeh
- Watermelon

Zinc is vital for pregnant women and is essential for the maintenance of the immune system. It may be sourced from:

- Legumes
- Nuts and seeds
- Grains
- Beans (kidney beans, garbanzo beans)

A good knowledge of food and their nutritional content is the key.

Chapter 3: How to Transition to a Vegan Diet

Transitioning from one diet to another is going to be a struggle. Abandoning old routines will not be easy, but a successful transition is truly impressive. In this chapter, you will learn how to take better control of your journey.

Transitioning Into Plant-based Foods

It seems simple, but you can ask anyone who has ever done it, and they will tell you that it is not. Making a change and adopting new habits can be very tricky, but it is not an impossibility.

The best way to tackle this is to follow a process. To make things simpler and more attainable, you will need a step-by-step plan of attack. For your journey to becoming a vegan, follow these steps to transition smoothly:

- **Step 1: Define your motivation.** Why are you making the transition? Are you doing this for health? Are you making an ethical choice for the environment and or for the welfare of animals? Do you want to lose weight? It is essential that this is clear because it will fuel your journey. If this is not adequately defined, it is quite easy to falter. But when there is a strong foundation established from the beginning, your transition will be backed up by a powerful motivation.

- **Step 2: Set your expectations.** It is not going to be a walk in the park. Whoever said it is going to be easy, probably did not go through the transition. It is tough, and you will want to quit, every time, so you have to be prepared. You have to be ready to be battling with yourself, the urges, the temptation, and so forth. Simply put, set your expectations realistically, but do not forget to remind yourself that it has been done before so you can do it too. Yes, it is hard, but there is a remarkable reward in the end.

- **Step 3: Educate yourself.** You cannot go through this without sitting down and studying it. The world of veganism is not something you do at a whim because there is so much to learn if you will do this right. It is more than just a knowledge of what to eat and what not to eat. This book sets you up at the right place, so take advantage of it.

- Step 4: Write down a plan. Armed with the right information, you can make things more attainable by writing down your ideas. It will serve as a guide so that you do not have to go through it like a headless chicken. A bonus chapter in this book includes a meal plan that you can use. It can be a template for the plan that you will write for yourself.

- Step 5: Take it one day at a time. Of course, all this physical and mental preparation will be for nothing without the corresponding action. If you are all set, then you have to make it happen. Just take it one day at a time. You do not have to hurry. If you fail one day, then you start all over again. Eventually, things will come naturally to you, and you will realize that veganism is already in your system.

Equipping Your Kitchen the Right Way

To launch your new lifestyle, you need to turn your kitchen into a vegan pantry. First you have to get rid of all the stuff that you do not need, throw it away or give it to someone; next you have to plan your meals; finally, you have to go shopping.

Shopping for food is going to be fun. As long as you know what to put into your shopping cart, it should not be so hard. As a beginner, you need to start with the basics. Eventually, you will build a vegan pantry that is fully-equipped.

Food	Sources
Butter Substitutes	oil and vegan butter
Carbohydrates	whole wheat pasta, soba noodles
Cheese Substitutes	nutritional yeast, rice cheese, soy cheese, nut and homemade vegan cheese
Condiments	Vegan mayonnaise, non-GMO mustard, and ketchup
Dairy Substitutes	almond yogurt, coconut yogurt, soy yogurt, vegan cream cheese
Egg Substitutes	applesauce and bananas, aquafaba, arrowroot eggs, chia seed eggs, chickpeas flour eggs, cornstarch eggs, ground flax seed eggs, tofu
Fruits	Any fruit in season especially those low in sugar such as grapefruit, lemon, cranberries, limes, pomegranate, strawberries, blueberries, blackcurrants

Milk Substitutes	almond milk, cashew milk, hemp milk, oat milk, rice milk, soy milk
Meat Substitutes	Field Roast sausages, Garden Fresh and Frozen Products, Sweet Earth
Nuts, Seeds and Dried Fruits	almonds, hemp seeds, chia seeds, ground flax seeds
Plant-Based Meat Substitutes	brown rice, bulgur, chickpeas, farro, legumes, organic non-GMO tofu, seitan, tempeh, quinoa, whole grains
Proteins	artichokes, asparagus, amaranth, almonds, beans, broccoli, black-eyed peas, chia seeds, chickpeas, edamame, green peas, green beans, hemp seeds, hemp milk, lentils, nutritional yeast, oatmeal, peanut butter, soy, spirulina, spinach, tahini, tofu, pumpkin seeds, quinoa

Seasonings	chili powder, cumin, dried basil, oregano, rosemary, and thyme, ground chipotle, ground ginger, onion powder, red pepper flakes, rice vinegar, sriracha, tamari or soy sauce,
Sweeteners	Blackstrap molasses, 100% organic maple syrup, unprocessed stevia, zulka
Vegetables	Anything in season. Leafy greens (most especially) But add a lot of parsley, garlic, cilantro, mint, and ginger (for flavoring)
Others	apple cider vinegar, chickpea flour, liquid smoke, olives, roasted red peppers, sundried tomatoes

Sticking to a Brand New Lifestyle

Once you successfully transition to veganism, your next goal is to maintain it. You have conquered the process, so it is necessary that you keep it in your system—otherwise, it will just be for nothing.

How can you stay vegan, now that you have already started? Here are some winning strategies you can apply:

- **Keep your head in the game.** Always remember your motivations and reasons, because it is supposed to give direction to your journey. If you want to keep going, you have to keep your head in the game.

- **Find joy in the eating vegan.** The mistake people make is they regard a diet like this as a "punishment." How can you find happiness, in punishment? You have to learn how to see the whole experience with a positive perspective. Explore the many amazing vegan recipes and allow yourself to enjoy the food selection. Healthy doesn't have to be boring. Vegan is not synonymous with bland. It can be magnificent.

- Pack your food. If dining out and going away is always a struggle for you, anticipate the worst. Instead of putting yourself in a wrong position, prepare for it. Pack your lunch to work, to trips, to meets, and so forth. Do not rely on the existence of a vegan menu. Instead, take matters into your own hands and pack your food.

- Find healthy substitutes. If you are afraid to indulge yourself with some of your cravings, then allow yourself tasty substitutes that will help bring happiness to your tummy.

- **Transition slowly.** Some people will consider going cold-turkey and abandon their old lifestyle to adopt an entirely vegan diet, but if you think this is going to be impossible, you can take it a pace that you can manage. Some people start by giving up on one animal product at a time until they become entirely vegan. You can begin with cutting on beef, or you can consider abandoning all meats except for seafood. Some people will start with one vegan meal per day until they are more confident about going completely vegan.

- **Add exercise.** If you want to give yourself room for some indulgence and you want to relax your diet, for a bit, add some physical activity that will keep things in control. This, in turn, will bring things in full circle because not only is your health consciousness focussed on the diet, but also the exercise.

Chapter 4: Avoiding These Common Mistakes

Your journey is not going to be an easy one, and you are bound to encounter problems along the way. Especially if you are not careful and you ignore the risks, things can go wrong.

As always, proper information is going to be your most potent weapon. If you take time to study veganism, it will be easier for you to avoid making mistakes.

Avoiding the Risks of Veganism

There are a few risks that you may encounter when you start the Vegan Diet:

1. *Eating too many calories.* Since rice, bread and noodles are non-animal, people tend to load up on these carbohydrates, so they end up eating so much more. As much as possible, concentrate on the vegetables and grains because they are the most nutritious. The mistake is that instead of becoming a vegetarian, one ends up being a starchatarian—and a diet like that is very high in calories.

2. *Eating too few calories.* Well, if you're not overeating, you may be eating too little. Vegetables are low in calorie, in general, and if your diet is concentrated on veggies, you may not supply your body efficiently. It, of course, will result in weakness and disease.

3. Not getting enough nutrients. You have to be realistic. Vegetables cannot solely sustain you, so you have to explore the world of veganism to be able to compensate your deficiency in protein, zinc, iron, calcium, Vitamin D, Vitamin B12 and omega-3 fatty acids. There are non-animal sources for these—and your knowledge is going to be important.

4. Drinking an insufficient amount of water. The body needs water (at least seven glasses a day), whether or not you are a vegan. But as one, water is necessary to move the fiber more efficiently. Your diet is going to be highly fibrous due to the fruits and vegetables, and you need water so that you can avoid problems with constipation, gas, and bloating.

5. **Putting little to no importance to meal planning.** Some people feel too confident, and so they abandon what they have been doing at the beginning of their journey, such as meal planning. That is fine really, but it makes you more prone to error. Meal planning allows you to be more exacting about your efforts. It guards your meals closely—so you can maintain the diet. As much as you can, religiously observe this habit so that you can check for nutrition, calories, and ingredients. Also, it is easier to ensure variety when you sit down to plan.

If you are not careful, it is easy to suffer from these risks, so make sure to pay more attention to what you are eating.

Writing Your Vegan Diet Plan

A sample plan is provided to you at the end of this book. You will use this plan as a template—so that you can begin to write your own. How do you write a diet plan?

- **Step 1: Know the boundaries of your diet.** What food can you eat? What food should you avoid? It is pertinent that you have this laid down before anything else because the next steps will rely on your perfect knowledge of the boundaries of your diet.

- **Step 2: Determine your macro ratios and calories.** How many calories will you be taking in on a daily basis? Is this going to be sufficient for your primary and special needs? Are you going to be working out? If so, you have to make sure that your caloric intake supports this. What is the ratio of your caloric macronutrients? How much will protein, fat, and carbohydrates your diet have? It is essential that you determine this so that you can design a meal plan that satisfies your body's demands and requirements.

- **Step 3: How many meals are you going to have per day?** Are you going to have three meals—breakfast, lunch, and dinner; or will you be having five meals—breakfast, lunch, dinner, am and pm snacks? You need to decide on this because you have to divide the macronutrients and calories accordingly.

- **Step 4: Create your menu.** If you are an expert in the kitchen and writing your recipes, you can have fun in this section of your plan writing because this is where you stretch your imagination and creativity. If you are clueless about forming a recipe, do not worry because there are too many sources that you can use. This book has included as much as 30 recipes for you to try. Feel free to tweak them according to your taste.

- **Step 5: Start shopping.** You have written down everything and have carefully planned it; now it is time for you to write down a shopping list based on your meal plan. A meal plan is good because it directs your actions in the grocery or market. You do not have to go from aisle to aisle thinking of what to get; you just have to follow a list based on the plan. It's going to be easy.

Nutritional Features of Your Vegan Diet

This book has talked about calories, nutritional macros and so forth. Perhaps you are confused about how to plan your diet. The following is a guide that you can use:

Caloric Macros (Macronutrients)

A person's daily caloric intake depends on this requirement. A person may supply himself with 1500-3000 calories depending on how active he is.

Gender	Age	Calories		
		Sedentary	Moderately Active	Active
Child	2-3	1000	1000-1400	1000-1400
Male	4-8	1400	1400-1600	1600-2000
	9-13	1800	1800-2200	2000-2600
	14-18	2200	2400-2800	2800-3200
	19-30	2400	2500-2800	3000
	31-50+	2200	2400-2600	2800-3000
	51 above	2000	2200-2400	2400-2800

Female	4-8	1200	1400-1600	1400-1800
	9-13	1600	1600-2000	1800-2200
	14-18	1800	2000	2400
	19-30	2000	2000-2200	2400
	31-50	1800	2000	2200
	51+	1600	1800	2000-2200

Your caloric macros are consist of protein, fat, and carbohydrates. The percentage that each one will take will depend on your personal need. Those who engage in a lot of physical activity will need increased amounts of carbohydrates for energy; those who follow the ketogenic diet will maintain a high fat, low carb diet; and those who support the paleo diet will keep a high protein, low carb diet.

- Protein contains 4 calories per gram.
- Carbohydrates contain 4 calories per gram.
- Fat contains 9 calories per gram.

The table above shows you an estimate of how much calories you need per day, depending on how active your life is. The most common percentage split for these macronutrients is 40:40:20 where 20% is fat. You can change the percentage depending on the type of diet you want to have but use this equation to compute for calories:

daily calorie intake x macro percentage = calories

This means that if you follow the macro split given above, your fat requirement per day (if you are a 30-year-old-female with a sedentary lifestyle) will be:

2000 x 0.2 = 400 calories

Since there are 9 calories per gram of fat, 400 / 9 = 44.44 grams. You need 44.44 grams of fat per day.

Now, here is a rundown of your nutrient requirements. It is essential that you supply your diet accordingly, to satisfy your body's needs.

Nutrient	Daily Requirement
Protein	0.9 g per kg weight
Iron	14.4-32.4 mg
Calcium	1000 mg (men and women between 19-50 years)
Vitamin B12	2 mcg
Vitamin D	800 IU
Iodine	150-300 mg
Zinc	15 mg
Omega-3 Fatty Acids	250-500 mg

There are also some applications that you can download on your smartphone and gadgets to be able to do this efficiently. Applications like "MyFitnessPal" helps you take a record of your meals and activities per day while accounting for calories and nutrition. The use of these apps will help ensure that you are getting everything you need.

Have you enjoyed this book so far? Hopefully, you have learned so much because you're already halfway--the next chapters will be even more exciting.

Chapter 5: Vegan Breakfast Recipes

The first meal of the day is vital. A lot of people tend to neglect it, but it is a very wrong practice. Your breakfast is meant to jumpstart your day to a good light, so make sure to have a good meal in the morning.

Check out these easy-to-follow recipes:

Chive Waffles with Soy Mushrooms and Maple

Serves: 6

Preparation: 25 minutes

Cooking: 20 minutes

Ingredients:

- 1 tbsp baking powder
- 130g flour
- 1 tsp lemon juice

- 1 tbsp maple syrup
- 500ml rice milk or soya milk
- 6 mushrooms, sliced
- 150g polenta
- 2 tsp light soy sauce
- 100g sweet potato, mashed
- 2 tbsp rapeseed oil
- bunch of chives snipped
- olive oil
- soya yogurt (optional)
- salt and pepper, to taste

Directions:

1. In a bowl, combine the milk, rapeseed oil and vinegar. Mix them well and add the sweet potato mash and blend everything well.
2. In another bowl, combine the flour, polenta, and baking powder. Season with salt. Combine the contents of both bowls then add the chives to finish the batter.
3. Preheat the waffle iron, then pour batter and cook for about 4-5 minutes.
4. In a small bowl, combine soy sauce with maple syrup. Coat the mushrooms with this mixture then season it with pepper. Finally, saute the mushrooms until they are cooked through.

5. Serve the mushrooms on top of the waffles, then add a dollop of soya yogurt and a sprinkle of chives.

Calories	Fat	Carbohydrates	Fiber	Protein	Sodium
227	8g	30g	4g	7g	1.2g

Avocado Salsa and Mexican Beans on Toast

Serves: 4

Preparation: 20 minutes

Cooking: 10 minutes

Ingredients:

- 1 avocado, finely sliced
- 2 cans black beans
- 4 slices bread
- 1 tsp chili flakes or 2 tsp chipotle paste
- 1 tsp ground cumin
- 2 garlic cloves, crushed
- ½ lime, juiced
- 4 tbsp olive oil
- 1 onion, finely chopped
- 270g cherry tomatoes, quartered
- bunch of coriander

Directions:

1. In a bowl, combine lime juice, ¼ onion, tomatoes, and 1 tbsp oil then set it aside.
2. In a skillet, saute remaining onions and the garlic, then add the cumin and chili flakes (or chipotle). Add a splash of water and the beans, then add most of the tomato mixture with most of the coriander.
3. Meanwhile, toast the bread with a drizzle of the remaining ¼ oil.
4. To serve everything, lay a scoop of the bean mixture on the toast and add a few slices of avocado, and top it with the remaining coriander and tomato mixture.

Calories	Fat	Carbohydrates	Fiber	Protein	Sodium
368	19g	30g	13g	12g	0.9g

Lemon Poppy Scones

Serves: 12

Preparation: 10 minutes

Cooking 15 minutes

Ingredients:

- 4 tsp baking powder
- 2 cups all-purpose flour
- 1 lemon, juiced and zested
- ¾ cup margarine
- 2 tbsp poppy seeds
- ½ tsp salt
- ½ cup soy milk
- ¾ cup white sugar
- ½ cup water

1. Preheat on to 400°F. Grease a baking sheet.
2. In a bowl, combine flour, baking powder, sugar, salt and sift them all together. Slowly add the margarine until the mixture is smooth.

3. Add the lemon juice and zest, poppy seeds, soy milk, and water. Mix everything to form the batter.
4. Spoon ¼ cup sized batter onto the baking sheet and make sure they are about 3 inches apart from each other.
5. Pop them into the oven and bake them for about 10-15 minutes or until they are golden.

Calories	Fat	Carbohydrates	Protein	Sodium
250	12.3	30.8g	3 g	0.354g

Vegan Crepes

Serves: 4

Preparation: 5 minutes

Cooking: 20 minutes

Ingredients:

- 1 cup unbleached all-purpose flour
- 2 tbsp maple syrup
- ½ cup soy margarine
- ½ cup soy milk
- ¼ tsp salt
- 1 tbsp turbinado sugar
- ½ cup water

1. In a large bowl, combine water, soy milk, ¼ cup margarine, maple syrup, sugar, flour, and salt. Cover everything and chill it in the refrigerator for about 2 hours.
2. In a skillet, heat soy margarine and pour about 3 tbsp of batter to create the crepe. Flip it to cook the other side.

3. You can choose any fresh fruits for your filling.

Calories	Fat	Carbohydrates	Protein	Sodium
268	12.1g	35.6g	4.3g	0.295g

Garbanzo-Oat Pancakes

Serves: 4

Preparation: 5 minutes

Cooking: 15 minutes

Ingredients:

- 1 tsp baking powder
- ½ tsp ground cinnamon
- ¼ cup yellow cornmeal
- ½ cup garbanzo bean flour
- ¾ cup rolled oats
- 1 cup water

Directions:

1. In a large bowl, combine oats, garbanzo bean flour, cinnamon, cornmeal and baking powder. You may add more water if the mixture is too thick. Mix everything continuously until it is smooth and creamy.
2. In a griddle, heat oil and drop a large spoonful of the batter to cook it. Let it cook for about 3 minutes per side.

3. Serve the pancakes with your favorite fresh fruits or syrup.

Calories	Fat	Carbohydrates	Protein	Sodium
133	1.9g	24.5g	4.9	0.125g

Chapter 6: Vegan Lunch Recipes

Lunch serves as a pit stop meal, so if you have a very hectic day, this meal is going to be very important. This is essential in ensuring that the body is not going to run out of supply to perform its various functions.

Check out these easy-to-follow recipes:

Seitan and Black Bean Stir-fry

Serves: 4

Preparation: 20 minutes

Cooking: 25 minutes

Ingredients:

- 1 can black beans
- 1 red chili, finely chopped
- 1 tbsp cornflour

- 1 tsp Chinese five-spice powder
- 3 garlic cloves
- 2-3 tbsp vegetable oil
- 300g pak choi, chopped
- 1 tbsp peanut butter
- 2 tbsp rice vinegar
- 1 red pepper, sliced
- 1 jar seitan pieces
- 2 spring onions, sliced
- 75g brown sugar
- 2 tbsp soy sauce
- rice or noodles, cooked

Directions:

1. In a food processor, combine the beans with the brown sugar, garlic, soy sauce, five-spice powder, rice vinegar, peanut butter and red chili. Add water to make it smoother, then pour everything into a saucepan and heat it until it thickens.
2. Dry the seitan then toss them into a bowl with cornflour then set it aside.

3. In a large pan, heat oil then stir-fry the seitan until it is brown on the edges, then set it aside.
4. Using the same pan, dry it and add oil. Saute the peppers, pak choi, spring onion and the remaining beans. Add the seitan and pour in the sauce. Bring everything to a boil and serve it on top of the cooked rice or noodles.

Calories	Fat	Carbohydrates	Fiber	Protein	Sodium
326	8g	37g	7g	22g	3.08g

Eggless Tofu Spinach Quiche

Serves 6

Preparation: 15 minutes

Cooking: 30 minutes

Ingredients:

- 2/3 cup dairy-free cheddar cheese, shredded
- ½ cup dairy free Swiss cheese, shredded
- 1 tsp garlic, minced
- 1/3 cup almond milk
- ¼ cup onion, diced
- 9-inch unbaked pie crust
- 10 oz frozen spinach, thawed and chopped
- 8 oz tofu
- salt and pepper, to taste

Directions:

1. Preheat oven to 350°F
2. In a blender, combine milk and tofu then blend it until smooth. Season with salt and pepper.
3. In a bowl, combine garlic, spinach, onion, swiss cheese, cheddar cheese and the prepared tofu mixture. Mix everything well and then pour it into the pie crust
4. Pop it into the oven and let it bake for 30 minutes or until the top is golden brown.

Calories	Fat	Carbohydrates	Protein	Sodium
288	18.8g	18.5g	12.7g	0.489g

Vegan Mac and No Cheese

Serves: 4

Preparation: 15 minutes

Cooking 45 minutes

Ingredients:

- 1 cup cashews
- 1 tsp garlic powder
- 1/3 lemon juice
- 1 tsp onion powder
- 1 onion, chopped
- 8 oz elbow macaroni
- 1/3 cup canola oil
- 1 tbsp vegetable oil
- 4 oz roasted red peppers
- 1 1/3 cups water
- 3 tbsp nutritional yeast
- salt, to taste

Directions:

1. Preheat oven to 350°F

2. In a pot, boil water with a pinch of salt and cook the macaroni to al dente, for about 8 to 10 minutes. Set it aside in a baking dish.
3. In a saucepan, heat oil and saute onions until browned and then add this to the macaroni.
4. In a blender, combine lemon juice, cashews, water, and salt. Slowly add the roasted red peppers, canola oil, garlic powder, nutritional yeast and onion powder. Continue mixing everything until you achieve a smooth consistency.
5. Add the mixture to the macaroni and pop the dish into the oven to bake for about 10 15 minutes or until it has browned.

Calories	Fat	Carbohydrates	Fiber	Protein	Sodium
648	31.2g	69.6g	1g	16.5g	0.329g

Tomato, Basil, and Olive Oil Pasta

Serves: 8

Preparation: 15 minutes

Cooking 10 minutes

Ingredients:

- ½ cup fresh basil, cut into strips
- 2 cloves garlic, minced
- ½ cup olive oil
- 16 oz farfalle pasta
- 2 Roma tomatoes, seeded and diced
- salt and pepper, to taste

Directions:

1. In a pot, boil water with salt and cook the pasta to al dente, for 8 to 10 minutes. Drain and set it aside.
2. In a bowl, toss the cooked pasta with olive oil, tomatoes, basil, and garlic. Season with salt and pepper and serve.

Calories	Fat	Carbohydrates	Protein	Sodium
345	14.9g	44.1g	8.4g	3g

Carrot Rice Nut Burger

Serves: 20

Preparation: 1 hour

Cooking: 1 hour 30 minutes

Ingredients:

- 1 cup cashews, toasted
- 6 carrots, chopped
- 1 tbsp extra virgin olive oil
- 1 sweet onion, chopped
- 3 cups brown rice, uncooked
- 1 lb unsalted sunflower seeds, toasted
- 6 cups water
- salt, to taste

Directions:

1. In a pot, boil rice in water and reduce heat to let it simmer for about 45 minutes
2. In a food processor, combine cashews, sunflower seeds and let it run until smooth. Set it aside.

3. Run the onions and carrots in the food processor until finely shredded and combine it with the nuts.
4. Run the rice with oil in the food processor until smooth and mix this with everything. Season with salt and form patties.
5. Grill the patties about 6-8 minutes per side or until they are browned. Serve with whole-wheat buns or salad greens.

Calories	Fat	Carbohydrates	Protein	Sodium
270	16.2g	26.3g	7.7g	0.073g

Chapter 7: Vegan Dinner Recipes

Dinners are more of a reward for whatever day you have had. It doesn't have to be heavy, but it should be nourishing enough to allow your body to recover from the day thoroughly. Some people would think to skip dinner because they're about to retire for the day. The body performs specific functions during sleep, so you need to supply it with what it needs, so it is renewed for the next morning.

Check out these easy-to-follow recipes:

Sweet Potato and Coconut Curry

Serves: 6

Preparation: 20 minutes

Cooking: 6 hours 30 minutes

Ingredients:

- 250g red cabbage, shredded
- ½ tsp cayenne pepper
- 2 red chilies, seeded and sliced
- 3 garlic cloves, crushed
- 1 small root ginger, peeled
- 400ml coconut milk
- 4 tsp olive oil
- 2 onions, sliced
- 300g passata
- 1 tsp paprika
- 2 tbsp peanut butter
- 2 red peppers, seeded and sliced
- 1 kg sweet potatoes, chopped
- bunch of coriander
- couscous, cooked

Directions:

1. In skillet, heat oil and saute onion and garlic until tender. Add the ginger, paprika, and cayenne. Cook everything for another minute and then put it into the slow cooker.
2. Using the same skillet, heat oil and saute the chili, red cabbage, and red pepper. Cook everything for about 4-5 minutes and then put it into the slow cooker.
3. Using the same skillet, add the remaining oil and fry the sweet potatoes until the edges have browned and then put it into the slow cooker.
4. Cover the contents of the slow cooker with coconut milk and passata. Cover everything and let it cook for about 6-8 hours or until the potatoes are tender.

5. Before finishing, add the peanut butter and season it with salt and pepper. Serve the curry on top of couscous and garnish it with coriander.

Calories	Fat	Carbohydrates	Fiber	Protein	Sodium
434	22g	47g	10g	6g	0.2g

Vegan Shepherd's Pie

Serves: 8

Preparation: 30 minutes

Cooking: 1 hour 20 minutes

Ingredients:

- 4 carrots, cubed
- 4 celery sticks, chopped
- 400g chickpeas
- 3 garlic cloves, crushed
- 2 leeks, chopped
- ½ small pack marjoram or oregano, roughly chopped
- 20ml olive oil
- 2 onions, chopped
- 1 small pack parsley, chopped
- 300g frozen peas
- 30g dried porcini mushrooms, soaked and drained
- 2 tsp smoked paprika
- 1.2kg potatoes
- ½ small pack sage, roughly chopped

- 300g frozen spinach
- 1 butternut squash, peeled and cubed
- ½ small pack thyme, picked
- 2 tbsp tomato puree
- 50ml vegetable oil
- 1 cube vegetable stock
- tomato ketchup (optional)

Directions:

1. Preheat oven to 350°F
2. In a saucepan, bring the unpeeled potatoes to a boil, until the skin separates. Drain and set it aside.
3. In a skillet, heat oil and saute onions, mushrooms, leeks, and carrots. Add vegetable stock and let things simmer.
4. Add garlic, paprika, tomato puree, squash and mixture of herbs. Finally, add the celery and cook everything.
5. Add the chickpeas, including the water in the can, then add the spinach and peas.

6. Peel the potatoes and mash 200g into the stock. Take the rest of the potatoes and combine it with olive oil and parsley.
7. Divide the potato filling into the pie dishes and top them with the chopped potatoes. Pop them into the oven and let it bake for 45 minutes or until the top is golden. Serve with or without ketchup.

Calories	Fat	Carbohydrates	Fiber	Protein	Sodium
348	11g	43g	13g	11g	0.5g

Roast Summer Vegetables and Chickpeas

Serves: 4

Preparation: 20 minutes

Cooking: 50 minutes

Ingredients:

- 1 aubergine, thickly sliced
- 400g can chickpeas
- 1 tbsp coriander seeds
- 1 bunch coriander, roughly chopped
- 3 courgettes, thickly sliced
- 3 garlic cloves, chopped
- 4 tbsp olive oil
- 1 onion, chopped
- 2 red peppers, seeded and chopped
- 2 potatoes, peeled and chopped
- 400g canned tomatoes, chopped

Directions:

1. Preheat oven to 428ºF
2. Take a roasting tin and put all the vegetables in it. Season it with coriander seeds, olive oil, salt, and pepper. Pop it into the oven and let it roast for about 45 minutes or until the vegetables turn brown on the edges.
3. Lower the heat and add the chickpeas and tomatoes, then let everything simmer. Drizzle with oil and add coriander just before you take it out of the heat.

Calories	Fat	Carbohydrates	Fiber	Protein	Sodium
327	15g	40g	9g	11g	0.51g

Veggies and Tofu in Peanut Sauce

Serves: 4

Preparation: 10 minutes

Cooking: 10 minutes

Ingredients:

- 1 head broccoli, chopped
- 1 ½ tbsp molasses
- 5 mushroom, sliced
- 1 red bell pepper
- 1 tbsp peanut oil
- ½ cup peanut butter
- 2 tbsp soy sauce
- 1 lb firm tofu, cubed
- 2 tbsp vinegar
- ½ cup hot water
- ground cayenne pepper, to taste

Directions:

1. In a skillet, saute red bell pepper, broccoli, mushroom, and tofu for about 5 minutes
2. Meanwhile in a bowl, combine hot water, peanut butter, soy sauce, vinegar, molasses, and cayenne pepper. Mix it well and pour this over the vegetables in the skillet. Let things simmer until the vegetables are tender.

Calories	Fat	Carbohydrates	Protein	Sodium
442	29.9g	24g	29g	0.641g

Vegan Fajitas

Serves: 6

Preparation: 20 minutes

Cooking: 20 minutes

Ingredients:

- 15 oz black beans
- 1 tsp chili powder
- 8.75 oz whole kernel corn
- ¼ cup, 2 tbsp olive oil
- 1 onion, sliced
- 1 tsp dried oregano
- 1 green bell pepper, julienned
- 1 red bell pepper, julienned
- 4 whole-wheat tortillas
- 1 tsp white sugar
- 2 yellow squash, julienned
- ¼ cup red wine vinegar
- 2 zucchini, julienned
- garlic salt, to taste
- salt and pepper, to taste

Directions:

1. In a bowl, combine vinegar, olive oil, chili powder, oregano, sugar, garlic salt, salt, and pepper. Mix everything well.
2. Add the yellow squash, zucchini, green pepper, red pepper, and onion. Let it marinate in the refrigerator for about 30 minutes. Drain the marinade before cooking.
3. In a skillet, saute the vegetables until they are tender. Add the beans and corn and continue cooking until the vegetables have browned.
4. Arrange the fajitas and stuff the filling into the tortillas to serve

Calories	Fat	Carbohydrates	Protein	Sodium
198	14.4g	17.9g	3g	0.130g

Chapter 8: Vegan Dessert Recipes

There is always room for dessert—and as a vegan, you should still make room for the sweet stuff because it is going to make meals so much more delightful. Do not think that just because you have turned vegan, you cannot enjoy the fun things in life. You are mistaken.

Check out these easy-to-follow recipes:

Vegan Carrot Cake

Serves: 12-15

Preparation: 35 minutes

Cooking: 25 minutes

Ingredients:

- 1 ½ tsp baking powder
- 4 carrots, grated

- 2 tbsp cashew nut butter
- 1 tsp cinnamon
- 4 sachets creamed coconut
- 250ml coconut oil, melted
- 420g plain flour
- 1 tsp ginger
- 1 tbsp lemon juice
- 1 tsp ground nutmeg
- 60ml, 210ml oat milk
- 1 orange, zest only
- 1 ½ tsp bicarbonate of soda
- 300g light brown sugar
- 50g icing sugar
- 1 ½ tsp vanilla essence
- 75g walnuts, chopped
- edible flowers, optional

Directions:

1. In a bowl, combine coconut cream with lemon juice and 2 tbsp hot water. Mix everything well until smooth, then add the cashew butter. Finally, add the icing sugar and once adequately mixed, set it aside in the refrigerator to set.
2. Preheat oven to 350°F. Grease two cake tins with coconut oil.
3. In a bowl, combine sugar and oil then add the milk and vanilla essence. Once mixed, add flour, bicarbonate of soda, baking powder, and orange zest. Lastly, add the carrots and nuts.
4. Divide the batter into the cake tins and pop them into the oven to bake for about 25-30 minutes or until a toothpick comes out cleanly.

5. Pile the cake on top of each other, with a layer of icing in the middle. Then spread the remaining frosting on top of the cake and finish it with a sprinkle of nuts, cinnamon, and edible flowers (if you are using).

Calories	Fat	Carbohydrates	Fiber	Protein	Sodium
501	31g	49g	2g	5g	0.45g

Salted Caramel Biscuit Bar

Makes: 18 pieces

Preparation: 45 minutes

Cooking: 15 minutes

Ingredients:

- 20g ground almonds
- 150g dairy-free dark chocolate
- 3 tbsp, 2 tbsp coconut oil, melted
- 125g Medjool dates pitted
- 50ml maple syrup
- ½ tbsp. almond milk
- 1 ½ tbsp. peanut butter or almond butter
- 80g porridge oats
- pinch of salt

Directions:

1. Preheat oven to 350°F and line a baking dish with parchment paper.
2. In a food processor, combine oats and let it run until flour-like. Add almonds, maple syrup and 3 tbsp coconut oil and mix everything well.
3. Once the batter is formed, roll it and then cut it into rectangular bars, then lay them on the baking sheet. Pop them into the oven and let it bake for about 10 minutes.
4. In the same food processor, combine the dates, peanut butter (or almond butter), coconut oil, and almond milk. Season this with salt and let everything run until it is smooth. One by one, dip the biscuits into the caramel mixture and set it aside.
5. In a heatproof bowl, melt the chocolate over a pan with hot water, making sure the water doesn't get into the chocolate. Dip the caramel dipped biscuits, then lay everything on the tray.

6. Pop the tray into the refrigerator and leave them inside until the chocolate has set.

Calories	Fat	Carbohydrates	Fiber	Protein	Sodium
137	8g	13g	2g	2g	0.1g

Mint-Chip Coconut Milk Ice Cream

Serves: 8

Preparation: 10 minutes

Ingredients:

- 1/3 cup agave syrup
- 3 oz vegan dark chocolate, chopped
- 24 fl oz coconut milk
- 1 tsp peppermint extract

Directions:

1. Chill all the ingredients to make the freezing process much quicker
2. In a blender, combine coconut milk, peppermint extract, and agave syrup. Run it until the mixture is smooth.

3. Following the manufacturer's instructions, transfer the contents to an ice cream maker. Add the chocolate and freeze everything for 2 hours before serving.

Calories	Fat	Carbohydrates	Protein	Sodium
269	22g	19.4g	2.3g	0.012g

Orange Vegan Cake

Serves: 16

Preparation: 15 minutes

Cooking 30 minutes

Ingredients:
- 1 ½ tsp baking soda
- 1 ½ cups all-purpose flour
- 1 orange, peeled
- 1 cup white sugar
- ½ cup vegetable oil
- ¼ tsp salt

Directions:
1. Preheat oven to 375°F, Grease an 8x8 baking pan
2. In a blender, combine orange until you measure 1 cup orange juice
3. In a bowl, combine blended orange juice, sugar, flour, baking soda, vegetable oil, and salt. Whish it well together and pour it into the baking pan.

4. Pop it into the oven and let it bake for 30 minutes or until cooked through and a toothpick comes out cleanly.

Calories	Fat	Carbohydrates	Fiber	Protein	Sodium
157	7g	22.8g	1g	1.3g	0.155g

Vegan Rose Meringues

Serves: 40

Preparation: 30 minutes

Cooking: 1 hour 30 minutes

Ingredients:

- ¾ cup aquafaba (chickpea water)
- ¼ tsp cream of tartar
- ¼ tsp lemon juice
- 1 tsp rose water
- ¾ cup confectioners' sugar

Directions:

1. Preheat oven to 200°F
2. In a large bowl, combine rose water, aquafaba, cream of tartar and lemon juice. Using an electric mixer, blend everything until it is light and fluffy. Add confectioner's sugar, by increments, until you form stiff peaks.
3. Scoop mixture into a piping bag and fit it with a round tip

4. Pipe mounds of the mixture on the baking sheets lined with baking sheets. Pop it into the oven and bake for 1 ½ to 2 hours or until the meringues are dry and firm.

Calories	Fat	Carbohydrates	Protein	Sodium
11	0g	2.4g	0g	0g

Chapter 9: Vegan Soups, Stews and Salads

Soups and salads are great appetizers or side dishes, so it's good to have them either as a small meal or as a filler. Stews, on the other hand, are a specialized type of dish that features a thick and flavorful sauce.

Crunchy Bulgur Salad

Serves: 4

Preparation: 10 minutes

Cooking: 15 minutes

Ingredients:

- 75g whole blanched almonds
- 200g bulgur wheat
- 150g frozen podded edamame (soya) beans
- 1 bunch of mint, finely chopped

- 3 tbsp extra virgin olive oil
- 2 oranges
- 1 bunch of parsley, finely chopped
- 2 romano peppers, seeded and sliced
- 150g radishes, finely sliced

Directions:

1. Cook the bulgur according to package instructions. Set it aside.
2. In a bowl, soak edamame in boiling water for a minute and then drain.
3. In a large bowl, combine the soaked edamame, almonds, radishes, peppers, parsley, and mint.
4. Peel 1 orange and cut them into segments. Add this to the bowl.

5. Juice the other orange and gather it in a small jar and combine it with oil. Season it and then shake it well to let it emulsify. Toss this over your salad.

Calories	Fat	Carbohydrates	Fiber	Protein	Sodium
483	22g	50g	9g	17g	0g

Tomato Soup

Serves: 4

Preparation: 15 minutes

Cooking: 20 minutes

Ingredients:

- 2 bay leaves
- 1 carrot, diced
- 1 celery stick, roughly chopped
- 2 tbsp olive oil
- 1 onion, diced
- 2 tsp tomato puree
- 1 pinch sugar
- 1 ¼ kg tomatoes, cored and quartered
- 1.2 liters vegetable stock
- salt and pepper, to taste
- sour cream (optional)

Directions:

1. In a pan, saute the onion, carrot, and celery. Cook all the vegetables until they are soft and have lost their color. Stir it continuously to avoid it sticking to the bottom of the pan.
2. Add the tomato puree and stir everything until the vegetables turn red.
3. Add the bay leaves and season everything with salt and pepper. Put a lid on the pan to allow the tomatoes to stew until they shrink.
4. Add the vegetable stock and cook until it boils then let it simmer. Remove from heat and let it stand. Remove the bay leaves and let the tomato soup run in the food processor until it is smooth.

5. Return to pan and heat. Season with salt and pepper to taste. You may serve this with chilled sour cream on top.

Calories	Fat	Carbohydrates	Fiber	Protein	Sodium
123	7g	13g	4g	4g	1.08g

Barley and Lentil Stew

Serves: 8

Preparation: 15 minutes

Cooking: 12 hours

Ingredients:

- ¾ cup pearl barley, uncooked
- 1 tsp dried basil
- 3 bay leaves
- 2 tsp garlic, minced
- ¾ cup dry lentils
- ¼ cup dried onion flakes
- 2 cups button mushrooms, sliced
- 1 oz shitake mushrooms, torn
- 2 tsp dried summer savory
- 2 quarts vegetable broth
- salt and pepper, to taste

Directions:

1. In a slow cooker, combine the vegetable broth, shitake mushrooms, button mushrooms, lentils, barley, garlic, onion flakes, summer savory, basil, bay leaves, salt, and pepper.
2. Cover and leave it to cook for about 4 to 6 hours. Remove bay leaves and serve.

Calories	Fat	Carbohydrates	Protein	Sodium
213	1.2g	43.9g	8.4g	0.466g

Spinach and Lentil Soup

Serves: 4

Preparation: 10 minutes

Cooking: 55 minutes

Ingredients:

- 1 tsp ground cumin
- 2 cloves garlic, crushed
- 3 cloves garlic, minced
- ½ cup lentils
- 2 white onions, sliced into rings
- 10 oz spinach
- 1 tbsp vegetable oil
- 2 cups water
- salt and pepper, to taste

1. In a pan, heat oil and saute onions until browned and add garlic, and saute for about a minute.
2. Add the water, and the lentils then bring everything to a boil. Reduce heat and let things simmer until the lentils soften.

3. Add spinach, cumin, and salt. Cover the pan again and let things simmer. Add the crushed garlic and pepper to taste.

Calories	Fat	Carbohydrates	Protein	Sodium
155	4.3g	24g	9.7g	0.639g

Black Bean and Corn Salad

Serves: 6

Preparation: 25 minutes

Ingredients:

- 1 avocado, peeled and diced
- 15 oz black beans
- ½ cup fresh cilantro, chopped
- 1 ½ cup frozen corn kernels
- 1 clove garlic, minced
- 1/3 cup fresh lime juice
- ½ cup olive oil
- 6 green onions, thinly sliced
- 1 red bell pepper, chopped
- 1/8 tsp ground cayenne pepper
- 1 tsp salt

Directions:

1. In a jar with lid, combine olive oil, lime juice, cayenne pepper, garlic, and salt. Cover and shake to combine all the ingredients
2. In a bowl, combine the corn, beans, bell pepper, avocado, tomatoes, cilantro and green onions. Toss everything well and pour the lime dressing over it. Toss the salad to coat the vegetables evenly.

Calories	Fat	Carbohydrates	Protein	Sodium
391	24.5g	35.1g	10.5g	0.830g

Chapter 10: Vegan Snack and Smoothie Recipe

Snacking can be very difficult. In between meals, you will feel slight hunger pangs, and everyone tends to grab a bag of chips or a bar of chocolate. As a transitioning vegan, it will be a challenge, so you have to equip yourself with excellent snacking ideas.

Check out these easy-to-follow recipes:

Strawberry and Oatmeal Smoothie

Serves: 2

Preparation: 10 minutes

Ingredients:

- 1 banana, chunks
- 1 cup almond milk
- ½ cup rolled oats

- 14 strawberries, frozen
- 1 ½ tsp agave nectar (optional)
- ½ tsp vanilla extract (optional)

Directions:

1. In a blender, combine oats, milk, banana, strawberries, vanilla extract and agave nectar and blend it. Run it until it is smooth and serve cold.

Calories	Fat	Carbohydrates	Protein	Sodium
205	2.9g	42.4g	4.2g	0.083 mg

Sweet Potato, Chili, and Peanut Butter Quesadillas

Serves: 2

Preparation: 15 minutes

Cooking: 45 minutes

Ingredients:

- 1 ripe avocado, peeled and chopped
- ½ pack coriander, torn
- ½ lime, juice and zest
- 3 tbsp olive oil
- 1 tbsp smoked paprika
- 2 tbsp crunchy peanut butter
- 3 sweet potatoes, thinly sliced
- 4 flour tortillas
- sriracha chili sauce, to taste

Directions:

1. Preheat oven to 400°F
2. In a roasting tin, combine sweet potatoes, 2 tbsp oil, and paprika and pop it in the oven for about 15 minutes or until the potatoes have become crisp.
3. In a bowl, combine avocado, lime zest and. Mash the avocados well, until it is smooth, and add the peanut butter and the remaining olive oil.
4. In a griddle pan, heat the tortillas on either side.
5. To arrange, lay the tortilla and spread the peanut butter mixture then add sweet potatoes and chili sauce. Add the other tortilla and press down to cook it even more. Flip the tortilla and do the same on the other side. Cut it into quarters and serve with lime wedges and crushed avocados.

Calories	Fat	Carbohydrates	Fiber	Protein	Sodium
947	51g	96g	18g	17g	1.7g

Raw Strawberry Jam

Makes: 1 350g jar

Preparation: 15 minutes

Ingredients:

- 2 tbsp chia seeds
- 2 tbsp lemon juice
- 2 tbsp maple syrup
- 400g strawberries, hulled

Directions:

1. In a food processor, blend ¾ strawberries and chop the rest.
2. Add the lemon juice, chia seeds and maple syrup. Stir well and then leave it for an hour to set. Stir it occasionally and wait for it to thicken.

3. Store it in a jar in the refrigerator for 4 days up to a month. Enjoy this on warm toast.

Calories	Fat	Carbohydrates	Fiber	Protein	Sodium
12	0.3g	2g	1g	0.2g	0g

Vegan Cashew Cream Cheese

Makes: 1 400g jar

Preparation: 15 minutes

Ingredients:

- 250g cashews
- 1 juice of lemon
- 2 tbsp nutritional yeast
- 1 tbsp water
- 1 bunch chives (optional)
- ½ tsp salt

Directions:

1. In a bowl, soak the cashews in water for 4 hours or overnight.
2. Drain water from the bowl and transfer the cashews to a food processor. Add lemon juice, nutritional yeast, salt, and water. Let things run until the mixture is smooth.
3. Transfer cream cheese mixture to a bowl and add chives. Store in the refrigerator for an hour and enjoy for as long as 3-4 days.

Calories	Fat	Carbohydrates	Fiber	Protein	Sodium
124	9g	4g	1g	5g	0.3g

Kale and Banana Smoothie

Serves: 1

Preparation: 5 minutes

Ingredients:

- 1 banana
- 1 tbsp flax seeds
- 2 cups kale, chopped
- 1 tsp maple syrup
- ½ cup light unsweetened soy milk

Directions:

1. In a blender, combine banana, flax seeds, kale, soy milk, and maple syrup. Blend it until smooth
2. Serve it over ice, or you can freeze the banana overnight

Calories	Fat	Carbohydrates	Protein	Sodium
311	7.3	56.6g	12.2g	0.110g

Bonus Chapter: 14-Day Vegan Getting Started Plan

Given what you have learned, it is now time for you to apply things and see how well you do. It is not going to be easy, making a switch, especially when it is too drastic. But here is a 14-day plan that you can use as a guide so that you can transition with more ease.

This two-week plan is only a starter, but use it as a template, so that you can fully launch your brand new lifestyle, with much ease.

WEEK 1

DAY	BREAKFAST	LUNCH	DINNER
MONDAY	Vegan Pancakes with Blueberries	Veggie Quesadillas	Ginger Noodles with Mixed Greens Salad
TUESDAY	Cinnamon Apple Oatmeal	Bean and Veggie Toast	Falafel Salad with Tahini Dressing
WEDNESDAY	English Muffin with Peanut Butter and Chia Berry Jam	Potato and Cauliflower Curry	Rainbow Veggie Spring Roll

THURSDAY	Kale and Spinach Smoothie	Stuffed Sweet Potatoes with Hummus	Barbecue-Style Portabello Mushrooms
FRIDAY	Oatmeal with Fresh Fruits and Nuts	Quinoa Pilaf	Chickpea Curry
SATURDAY	Yogurt with Muesli and Mixed Berries	Tomato and Non-Dairy Cheddar Cheese Toast	Mozzarella, Zucchini and Basil Frittata
SUNDAY	Healthy Green Smoothie	Chickpea Salad Roll	Lentil Artichoke Stew

WEEK 2

DAY	BREAKFAST	LUNCH	DINNER
MONDAY	Oatmeal Banana Bites	Balsamic Zucchini Sandwich	Roasted Vegetable Lettuce Wraps
TUESDAY	Strawberry and Oatmeal Breakfast Smoothie	Stir-fry Yam and Bok Choy on Brown Rice	Black Bean Quinoa Bowl
WEDNESDAY	Avocado and Egg on Toast	Edamame Greek Salad	Sweet Potato and Lentil Chilli

THURSDAY	Quinoa Cereal with Almond Milk	Apple and Cheese Pita Pocket	Cashew and Vegetable Stir-fry	
FRIDAY	Peanut Butter and Cinnamon Toast	Veggie Fajitas	Vegetarian Pita Pizza	
SATURDAY	Loaded Breakfast Burritos	Artichoke and Tomato Gnocchi	Butternut Squash and Black Bean Tostadas	
SUNDAY	Cornbread Muffins with Assorted Berries	Chickpea Salad with Roasted Red Pepper Hummus Dressing	Carrot and Red Pepper Soup with Toasted Whole-Wheat Tortillas	

Final Words

Thank you again for purchasing this book! I really hope this book is able to help you.

The next step is for you to join our email newsletter to receive updates on any upcoming new book releases or promotions. You can sign-up for free and as a bonus, you will also receive our "*7 Fitness Mistakes You Don't Know You're Making*" book! This bonus book breaks down many of the most common fitness mistakes and will demystify many of the complexities and science of getting into shape. Having all this fitness knowledge and science organized into an actionable step-by-step book will help you get started in the right direction in your fitness journey! To join our free email newsletter and grab your free book, please visit the link and signup: www.hmwpublishing.com/gift

Finally, if you enjoyed this book, then I would like to ask you for a favor, would you be kind enough to leave a review for this book? It would be greatly appreciated!

Thank you and good luck in your journey!

Plant-Based

Diet

The Ultimate Beginner's to Plant Based Diet Guide & Recipes for Beginners - Improve Your Health, Get More Energized and Feel Your Best + 50 Easy & Delicious Recipes

By *Jennifer Louissa*

For more great books visit:

HMWPublishing.com

Get another book for Free

I want to thank you for purchasing this book and offer you another book (just as long and valuable as this book), "Health & Fitness Mistakes You Don't Know You're Making", completely free.

Visit the link below to signup and receive it:

www.hmwpublishing.com/gift

In this book, I will break down the most common health & fitness mistakes, you are probably committing right now, and I will reveal how you can easily get in the best shape of your life!

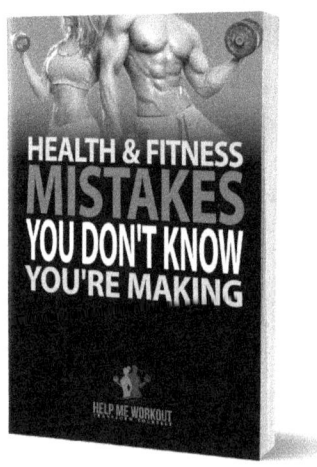

In addition to this valuable gift, you will also have an opportunity to get our new books for free, enter giveaways, and receive other valuable emails from me. Again, visit the link to sign up:

www.hmwpublishing.com/gift

Table Of Contents

Introduction 13

Chapter 1: Discovering the Riches of Plant-Based Food 16

    Achieve Your Full Health Potential 16

    Iron 19

    Calcium 23

    Vitamin D 28

    Be Fit and Strong 30

    Gain Energy and the Best Nutrients 33

    Peanut Butter, Banana, Cranberry Smoothie (serves 1) 41

    Mango Smoothie Bowl (serves 1) 41

    Golden Glow Smoothie (serves 1) 42

    Minty Cucumber-Apple Smoothie 43

    Alkaline Booster Smoothie 43

    High Dietary Fiber 45

Vitamin C 46

Magnesium 47

Potassium 47

Develop the Right Diet Practices 49

Key Takeaways 51

Chapter 2: Implementing the Plant-Based Diet at Home 53

Master the Grocery Basics 53

Fruit Items 54

Vegetable Items 55

Legumes 55

Whole Grains 55

Substituting Dairy Products 56

Prepare Your Kitchen Kingdom 57

Pressure Cooking 58

Slicing and Chopping 58

Bowls 59

Blending 59

Food Processing 59

Create the Right Plant Based Adaptations 60

Ensuring Vitamin B12 60

Ensuring Necessary Fatty Acids 61

Preventing Anemia 61

Ensuring Protein 62

Minimizing Meat 62

Nail the Keys to a Disciplined Diet 63

Step 1: There are no pressures. 64

Step 2: Aim for the mini-goals. 65

Step 3: Initiatives are the real actions. 65

Step 4: Find delight in the variety of plant-based food options. 66

Step 5: Room for a healthy break is available 67

Step 6: Reinforce nutritious eating with other healthy practices. 68

Step 7: More review and education equates to more motivation. 70

Step 8: Go for a Plant-Based Diet with friends. 71

Key Takeaways..72

Chapter 3: Becoming a Role Model of Nutrition 75

Access the Advantages of Understanding Nutrition Facts...75

Body Mass Index 76

Calories 77

Carbohydrates..79

Sugars 80

Protein 82

Fat 85

Vitamins 86

Minerals 87

Water 90

Chapter 4: Begin the Day with Plant-Based Breakfasts 93

Oats to Love 93

Granola Energizer 96

The Pancake Solution 99

The Energy Porridge 102

Start the Day with Salad 105

Rich Rice Pudding 109

Merry to Eat Muffins 111

Quick Quinoa for a Busy Day 113

A Delightful Chickpea Omelet Plate 115

Fabulous Fruit Tart 118

Chapter 5: Love Lunch Pack Solutions 122

The Most Desirable Chili Bowl 122

Plant-Based Meatloaf 127

Curried Potatoes in Thai Style 131

Perfect Pineapple Fried Rice 134

A Valuable Vegetable Quiche 137

Lasagna for my Lunchbox 141

A Triple-B Burger 144

An Enchanting Enchilada Dish 147

Tasty Tofu 150

A Vegetable Wrap Wonder 152

Chapter 6: Dig in with Plant Based Dinners 155

Vietnamese Noodles for the Soul 155

Effortlessly Made Pizza 160

Cobbler Crave Creator 163

Plant-Based Casserole 166

A Surprising Stew 171

A Tempeh Treat 174

Oh My! Bulgur Pilaf! 177

Sweet Potatoes and Kale from Africa 180

A Nutritious Pasta Plate 183

The Best Brown Rice Sushi 187

Chapter 7: Sweet Find Snacks 192

Burrito Bites 192

Healthy Hummus 195

Fruity Quesadilla 198

Veggie Poppers to Adore 200

Amazing Asparagus Quick Eat 204

A Quick Apple Delight 207

Break Time Crunch Rolls 209

Creative Cookies 212

Great Guacamole 215

Bright Banana Mash 217

Chapter 8: Divine Desserts 219

Carrot Cake to Go 219

Cool Strawberry Cupcakes........................223

Must-Have Gingerbread 226

Fabulous Fruit Squares 230

Colorful Parfait 234

Precious Pudding..238

Mouthwatering Chocolate Gelato 240

Datable Dates...242

Pretty Pumpkin Pie....................................245

Berry Tempting Tarts 248

Chapter 9: The 14-Day Getting Started Meal Plan 251

Understand Planning is Vital 251

2 Weeks of Plant-Based Dishes 255

Week 1...255

Week 2 259

Establish Success with Your Health Goals 262

- Educate Yourself 263
- Focus on Crowding Out, Not Cutting Out...264
- Find Creative Plant-Based Recipes to Inspire You.....................................265
- Focus on the Basics........................266
- Take it One Step at a Time............267
- Stick to Whole Foods 268
- Consume a Wide Variety of Plant-Based Food 268

Final Words...270

About the Co-Author........................272

Introduction

The Plant-Based Diet is a favourite food plan that is getting more and more attention. It is known to be a successful diet that genuinely develops your full health potential. You will benefit having *The Ultimate Beginner's Guide to the Plant-Based Diet* because it will provide all the information needed on this amazing healthy eating habit and lifestyle.

This book that will always come in handy when you want to establish nutritious eating habits because it is composed of delightful features such as:

- Plant-based diet practices that will help improve your health

- Information on food that provides you more energy

- Health strategies that will make you feel and be at your best

- Recipes that are nutritious and easy to prepare

- A 14-Day plant-based meal plan that is healthy and delicious

Furthermore, this guide aims to achieve the following objectives:

1. Differentiate the Plant-Based Diet from other diets

2. Identify the plant-based food choices and offer 50 plant-based recipes

3. Elaborate on the methods when following a plant-based diet

4. Emphasize the value of a menu rich in whole foods towards a healthy and energetic lifestyle

I sincerely hope you enjoy the reliable information that this book will offer you.

Also, before you get started, I recommend you **joining our email newsletter** to receive updates on any upcoming new book releases or promotions. You can sign-up for free, and as a bonus, you will receive a free gift. Our "*Health & Fitness Mistakes You Don't Know You're Making*" book! This book has been written to demystify, expose the top do's and don'ts and to finally equip you with the information you need to get in the best shape of your life. Due to the overwhelming amount of misinformation and lies told by magazines and self-proclaimed "gurus", it's becoming harder and harder to get reliable information to get in shape. As opposed to having to go through dozens of biased, unreliable and un-trustworthy sources to get your health & fitness information. Everything you need to help you has been broken down in this book for you to easily follow and to immediately get results to achieve your desired fitness goals in the shortest amount of time.

Once again, to join our free email newsletter and to receive a free copy of this valuable book, please visit the link and signup now: www.hmwpublishing.com/gift

Chapter 1: Discovering the Riches of Plant-Based Food

Learning about the plant-based diet can be an enriching experience. This food plan provides several health benefits that can help you achieve your nutrition goals. As you read this chapter, you will discover these advantages and more valuable facts on this great diet.

Achieve Your Full Health Potential

First, you are probably wondering: What is this diet all about and how does it work?

This healthy eating habit is about eating whole fruits and vegetables as well as avoiding or limiting eating animal-based food. The term "whole" refers to food grown from the farm, trees, and bushes, excluding excludes plant fragments or processed plants. Therefore, the food plan is also known as the Whole Food Plant-Based (WFPB) diet.

Currently, many people are practicing or trying out consuming a diet consisting of whole foods because it is believed to be an efficient way to achieve and maintain one's full health potential. Health experts strongly recommend this food plan because it helps:

- Strengthen the body
- Reboots energy
- Provide good nutrients
- Prevent common illness and disease conditions

The diet comprises of the following:

- Fruits
- Vegetables
- Legumes
- Tubers
- Whole grains

Some plant-based diet minimizes eating animal-based food choices and plant fragments. Others eliminate these food choices from their meal plans. Animal-based food choices include meat, dairy products, fish, and eggs. As mentioned earlier, plant fragments are processed plants. Some examples are juiced fruits, fruit pies, and syrups. The diet limits these food picks because they are most likely to trigger health risks.

You may also be wondering: What are the disadvantages of eating mostly fruits and vegetables? According to Tuso, P.J, MD, Ismail, M.H, MD, Ha, B.P, MD, and Bartolotto, C., MA, RD (2013) of The Permanente Journal, this healthy diet is a recommendable food plan to prevent conditions of common illnesses and diseases. Patients with diabetes, obesity issues, high blood pressure, and cardiovascular disease can significantly benefit from this diet. But the health experts also note the few risks you may face in this eating plan.

First among the disadvantages is you may suffer from deficient in Vitamin B12. This vitamin is necessary for blood formation and cell division. It is essential to add food choices with this nutrient in your meal plan. You may also have inefficient intakes of healthy fatty acids such as omega-3 fatty acids. You can ensure you have these necessary fatty acids by adding walnuts in your menu and cooking with canola oil.

Iron

Health expert's stress that claims about the reduced amount of iron in the body, leading to iron deficiency anemia is not true. Anemia develops when there is an insufficient amount of healthy haemoglobin in the red blood cells of the body. Haemoglobin is a protein molecule whose primary role is to carry oxygen from the lungs and then transport it to every cell and tissue, and then carry carbon dioxide from the cells and tissues back to the lungs. With an insufficient supply of iron, the body cannot produce enough haemoglobin. Thus, the body does not get sufficient amount of oxygen that it needs and is unable to remove carbon dioxide from the body to be exhaled.

Iron deficiency and anemia is not a problem in plant-based diets. When you follow the principles, consume plants rich in iron, and follow the absorption principles, it is not hard to get enough iron, whether you are just reducing or eliminating animal-based foods. Consume more foods that are rich in iron, such as the following:

- Legumes: lima beans, tempeh, tofu (2.15 mg per quarter of serving block), soybeans, lentils, kidney beans (3.93 mg/cup)

- Whole grains: oatmeal, brown rice, fortified cereals, quinoa (2.76 mg/per serving cup), barley, bulgur, millet, buckwheat

- Seeds and Nuts: unhulled sesame (1.31 mg/tablespoon), cashews (8.22 mg/cup), sunflower, pistachio (5 mg/cup), pine, squash, pumpkin (2.12 mg/cup), macadamia (5 mg/cup), squash 2.12 mg/cup), almonds (5.32 mg/cup)

- Vegetables: Tomato sauce

- Others: prune juice, blackstrap molasses (2.39 mg per 2 teaspoons)

- Dark Leafy Greens: Spinach (6.43 mg iron per 1 cup of cooked amount), collard greens, turnip greens, kale, Swiss Chard (3.95 mg/cup of cooked amount), beet greens (2.74 mg/cup of cooked amount)

- Spirulina (2mg per 2 tablespoons)

- Dried fruit: peach halves (6.50 mg/cup), prunes, apricots, raisins

- Dark powder and chocolate (contains 10.12 milligrams iron per 3 ounces of 70-80% of dark chocolate

Likewise, consuming iron from plants with vitamin C helps increase the absorption of iron up to as much as 5 times more, such as eating rice and beans with salsa, falafel with tomatoes. The iron in seeds, grains, and beans is better when combined with the vitamin C in vegetables and fruits. You can pair dark chocolate with oranges. Moreover, some iron-containing plants also contain vitamin C, such as tomato sauce, broccoli, and leafy greens.

You should also avoid tea and coffee when consuming high iron meals. These drinks, along with other beverages that contain tannins, that prevent the absorption of iron. Drink them 1 hour before or 2 hours after a meal.

Finally, less is better. Taking a 15-mg pill of iron a day does not mean your body absorbs all the 15 milligrams. The body absorbs less iron when you take a higher amount of iron on a one-time intake. However, consuming iron by smaller amounts throughout the day increases absorption. The recommended daily intake is as follows:

Age	Female	Male	Lactation	Pregnancy
Birth - 6 months old	0.27 milligrams	0.27 milligrams		

7 to 12 months old	11 milligrams	11 milligrams		
1 to 3 years old	7 milligrams	7 milligrams		
4 to 8 years old	10 milligrams	10 milligrams		
9 to 13 years old	8 milligrams	8 milligrams		
14 to 18 years old	15 milligrams	11 milligrams	10 milligrams	27 milligrams
19 to 50 years old	18 milligrams	8 milligrams	9 milligrams	27 milligrams
51 years old and above	8 milligrams	8 milligrams		

Calcium

However, the calcium content of plants depends on

the available calcium that they can absorb from the soil. Plants grown in bone meal or lime-treated soil will have high calcium content. Moreover, these results were obtained from hydroponically grown plants, which have higher calcium content than field-grown plants because they absorb calcium from the nutrient solution in a hydroponic system.

You should also reduce the amount of salt you add to your dishes. The same study revealed that too much salt leads to excessive calcium excretion via urine since both salt and calcium share some of the same transport systems. Each 2300 mg sodium excreted by the kidney pulls 40 to 60 mg of calcium from the body, which over time can lead to various calcium deficiency related diseases, such as osteoporosis or bone disease.

You also need to reduce your intake of dietary protein, as well as amino acids, because high amounts minimize the absorption of calcium and increase excretion.

Caffeine also affects calcium levels in the body.

However, it is negligible. An average cup or 240 ml of coffee decreases calcium by 2 to 3 milligrams. On the other hand, if you are not getting enough calcium from the foods you are eating, it might be best to avoid caffeine.

So if you are eliminating animal-based foods from your diet, you need to take a calcium supplement to meet your daily need. The recommended daily intake is as follows:

- Tofu with calcium = 80 mg per 126 grams

- Kale = 30.1 mg per 85 grams

- Fruit punch with calcium citrate malate = 156 mg/ 240 ml or 1 cup

- Broccoli = 21.5 mg per 71 grams

- Bok choy = 42.5 mg per 85 grams

- White beans = 24.7 mg per 110 grams

- Chinese cabbage flower leaves = 94.7 mg per 65 grams

- Chinese mustard greens = 85.3 mg per 85

grams

- Pinto beans = 11.9 mg per 86 grams

- Red beans 9.9 mg per 172 grams

However, calcium content of plants depends on the available calcium that they can absorb from the soil. Plants grown in bone meal or lime-treated soil will have high calcium content. Moreover, these results were obtained from hydroponically grown plants, which have higher calcium content than field-grown plants because they absorb calcium from the nutrient solution in a hydroponic system.

You should also reduce the amount of salt you add to your dishes. The same study revealed that too much salt leads to excessive calcium excretion via urine since both salt and calcium share some of the same transport systems. Each 2300 mg sodium excreted by the kidney pulls 40 to 60 mg of calcium from the body, which over time can lead to various calcium deficiency related diseases, such as osteoporosis or bone disease.

You also need to minimize your intake of dietary protein because of high amounts of it, as well as amino acids, reduces the absorption of calcium and increases excretion.

Caffeine also affects calcium levels in the body. However, it is negligible. An average cup or 240 ml of coffee decreases calcium by 2 to 3 milligrams. On the other hand, if you are not getting enough calcium from the foods you are eating, it might be best to avoid caffeine.

So if you are eliminating animal-based foods from your diet, you need to take a calcium supplement to meet your daily need. The recommended daily intake is as follows:

- **Children 1 to 3 years old:** 700 milligrams

- **Children 4 to 8 years old:** 1,000 milligrams

- **Children 9 to 18 years old:** 1,300

milligrams

- **Adults 19 to 50 years old:** 1,000 milligrams
- **Women 51 to 70 years old:** 1,200 milligrams
- **Men 51 to 70 years old:** 1,000 milligrams
- **Men and Women 71 years old and above:** 1,200 mg

Vitamin D

On the other hand, vitamin D is vital because it helps regulate the metabolism of calcium, as well as the immune system and the gut function, protect the body from specific forms of cancer, promotes healthy mood, and reduces inflammation. It is primarily found in seafood, dairy products, eggs, and organ meats.

An insufficient amount of vitamin D causes

osteoporosis and other bone problems, depression, and decreased colon health.

To get your daily-recommended intake, get a good dose of sunshine for at least 15 minutes. Sunlight is the best source of vitamin D, hence referred to as the sunshine vitamin. Mushrooms are an excellent source. A cup contains 2 IU or 1 percent of your daily intake. For example, dried shiitake mushrooms contain 154 IUs of vitamin D per 3 ounces of serving, morel mushrooms contain 212 IUs per 3 ounces serving, and mushrooms treated with natural light can provide as much as 600 IUs per 3 ounces of serving, such as Monterey sliced baby bellas. Two cups of non-dairy yogurt and milk is also a good source. You can also take D2 supplement also called ergocalciferol, an animal-free supplement for vitamin D. It is obtained from yeast and is effective as vitamin D3, which are animal derived vitamin D supplements. However, vitamin D2 levels drop quickly after a couple of days compared to vitamin D3. Taking vitamin D2 pills a day ensures you get the amount close to the daily-recommended intake. Vegan vitamin D3 is now also available, which is more absorbable than D2 in the blood.

Knowing the pros and cons of this diet can help you adapt its practices according to your needs. It also helps when you want to share the diet's riches with your family and friends. Most importantly, your full health potential will become more attainable.

Be Fit and Strong

Achieving full health potential is the big picture that you willingly take on. Dieters succeed because of tiny, yet essential details of this vision are very motivating. One of the small benefits is the fact that the plant-based diet makes you achieve your ideal body fitness and helps you become strong.

Health researchers of the Nutrition & Diabetes journal proved that this healthy eating habit could be a tool for a healthy and fit body through a recent experiment. The researchers asked 23 patients in the age range of 35-70 years old to practice and follow the WFPB diet for three months. The eating plan had no energy supplement restrictions and had additional sources of Vitamin B12. The patients were known diagnosed cases of obesity with hypertension, type 2 diabetes, hypercholesterolemia, and ischemic heart disease. The health professionals concluded there was a substantial difference in cholesterol and body mass index (BMI). The patients achieved more significant weight loss compared to other dietary practices.

McMacken, M. and Shah, S. (2017) of the Journal of Geriatric Cardiology state that a diet high in fruits and vegetables play a minor role in preventing type 2 diabetes. It is more valuable in increasing fiber and phytonutrients, decreasing saturated fats, and promoting good body weight among several other health benefits.

It is evident that health experts believe that the plant-based diet can be a crucial element in developing and maintaining a fit body.

Their research highlights that a healthy eating habit rich in whole foods give you the following benefits:

- Being effective with necessary weight loss
- Reducing migraines and proper BMI maintenance
- Reducing allergies
- Preventing common illnesses and diseases
- Promising longer life

Getting your body molded to be healthy and fit is a definite objective you can attain now that you know that the plant-based diet can help you. This rich characteristic of the benefit secures your health. Once you begin with the food plan, you will notice progress slowly. You will witness and feel that your body's health is better than it ever was before.

Gain Energy and the Best Nutrients

Gaining energy and the best nutrients are other motivating small benefits that give plant-diet takers full health potential.

Plant-based dieters are more energetic than animal-based eaters because they include the right food choices in their eating plan. Many plant eaters do this procedure:

1. Create food plans that provide their daily energy need, making shopping and cooking preparation easier.

2. Invest in time for preparing ingredients for energy dishes. Experts believe that you can spend a minimum of 45 minutes weekly with vegetables.

3. Eat breakfasts with complex carbohydrates, including in fruits, vegetables, and whole grains. They help give your body energy that starts your day right.

4. Drink plant-based smoothies and replace coffee with fruit. With or without plant protein powder, plant-based smoothies give both energy and nutrients. Fruit can also be considered a better energy source than coffee because Vitamin C from fruits offers energy sustainment.

Smoothies are an excellent option for breakfast or snack. They only need a couple of ingredients, they are very easy to make, and they can be made to be a grab-and-go meal. Just prepare them ahead of time and grab them out of the fridge during a busy day. You can blend a smoothies and then freeze it. Just defrost in the refrigerator overnight before drinking.

You can also prepare the ingredients, pack them in quart bags or canning jars, label the containers with the name of the smoothie and date it was packed and then freeze. When labeling, be specific. Write how much liquid is needed and add what boosters you want to add and how much. When ready to enjoy a smoothie, just keep it on the counter for a couple of minutes or put in warm water and then blend until smooth. These pre-packed blends are good for a couple of months, but they are best when you make them into a smoothie within 2 to 4 weeks.

They are rich blends of fruits, vegetables, and a liquid base, plus some boosters and thickeners. Others add non-leafy vegetables and herbs into the mix for added health benefits.

These super nutritious drinks are packed with vitamins, minerals, phytonutrients, antioxidants, and much more. Most of the time, they do not contain any artificial sweeteners and are low in bad fat and calories. The combination of fresh ingredients enhances metabolism that aid weight loss, detoxify the body, helping flush out wastes and toxins, and boosts immunity, keeping your body healthy.

These fast food blends will undoubtedly make a perfect addition to your plant-based diet. Depending on your taste buds and needs, you can mix and match your favorite vegetables and fruits. Here is a simple guide to the leafy greens, liquid, fruits, vegetables, thickeners, and boosters that you can blend. Once you find the perfect ratio of the ingredients, they won't taste green.

Leafy Greens and/or Herbs (1 cup)	Liquids (1 cup)	Fruits and/or Vegetables (1 1/2 cup)	Thickeners	Boosters

Basil	Almond Milk	Apple	Avocado	Healthy fats, such as coconut oil, flaxseed oil, avocado, and cashews
Bok Choy	Coconut Milk	Avocado	Unsweetened Nut Butter	
Cilantro	Coconut Water	Banana	Yogurt	
Collards	Water	Beets		
Dandelion		Berries		
Dill		Grapes		Protein: nuts and seeds, such as chia seeds, sesame seeds, cashews, and pistachios, OR protein powder, such as hemp protein, soy protein, brown rice protein, and pea protein
Kale		Jicama		
Lavender		Mango		
Mint		Orange		
Parsley		Peach		
Romaine		Pear		
Rosemary		Pineapple		
Sage		Snow Peas		
Spinach		Squash		
Swiss Chard		Sunchokes		
Tarragon		Sweet Potatoes		
Thyme		Tomatoes		
		Zucchini		

Because these smoothies contain fruits, they can already be sweet. But you can add Medjool dates, coconut water, coconut sugar, cinnamon, blackstrap molasses, goji berries, pure maple syrup, or lucuma powder to sweeten the blend. You can also add flavourings, such as cocoa powder, shredded coconut, nutmeg, cinnamon, or vanilla extract.

Important Reminder:

Whether you are adding greens to your smoothies or adding them to your dishes, eating the same leafy green can cause "alkaloid build-up." All raw leafy greens contain small amounts of toxins to protect them from being consumed by animals and wiping their species. If you use the same leafy green every day for several weeks, the toxins can build up in your body, causing symptoms of alkaloid build-up, such as nausea, tingling in the fingertips, and fatigue. There is no need to be alarmed, toxin build-up is rare and if you experience any symptoms, they will be mild and will not last long. However, it is always better to be safe.

Use a variety of leafy greens for your plant-based smoothies and raw dishes. Rotate them weekly and use leafy greens from different family groups. Greens from different family contain different toxins, so if you switch a leafy green from one family to another from a different family, it will prevent alkaloid build-up. For example, you can buy kale and spinach for this week, and then buy romaine lettuce and Swiss chard for next week.

Here is a simple guide to the greens that you can swap.

Crucifers	Amaranth	Asteraceae	Apiaceae
Kale	Spinach	Dandelion	Celery
Arugula	Beet greens	Romaine lettuce	Cilantro
Collard greens	Chard		Carrot tops
Cabbage			
Bok Choy			

Here are a couple of smoothies that you can enjoy. To blend, just add the liquid and the fruits and vegetables first, blend, and then combine the other ingredients. Add any sweetener, or flavoring of your choice, and blend. If you want a thicker smoothie, then you can add ice after and then mix again. For a cold beverage without any ice, use frozen fruits and vegetables.

Peanut Butter, Banana, Cranberry Smoothie (serves 1)

- 1 1/2 tablespoon ground hemp seeds,
- 1 cup unsweetened coconut milk
- 1 heaping tablespoon (closer to 2 tablespoons) unsweetened smooth organic peanut butter
- 1 large-sized organic banana, sliced and then frozen
- 1 tablespoon ground chia seeds
- 1/4 cup dried organic cranberries (sweetened with fruit juice or unsweetened)
- 3-4 ice cubes

Mango Smoothie Bowl (serves 1)

- 1 bananas

- 1/2 cup mango, diced
- 3 handfuls baby kale {or spinach}
- 2 tablespoons hemp seeds
- 1/2 cup unsweetened almond milk {or preferred milk}
- 1/8 teaspoon pink salt {or sea salt}
- Handful ice

For toppings:

- Sliced mango
- Drizzle of preferred liquid sweetener
- Red Russian kale sprouts
- Hemp seeds

Golden Glow Smoothie (serves 1)

- 1 cup orange juice, freshly squeezed
- 1 sweet apple, organic, peeled and chopped

- 1 teaspoon ginger, fresh grated
- 1/2 cup baby spinach
- 5 ice cubes

Minty Cucumber-Apple Smoothie

- 6 mint leaves
- 1/2 cucumber, sliced
- 1 green apple, organic, peeled and chopped
- 1/2 cup cold purified water
- 5 ice cubes
-

Alkaline Booster Smoothie

- 2 tablespoons almond butter or coconut oil
- 1/4 cup coconut water
- 1/4 avocado

- 1/2 pear

- 1 teaspoon chia seeds

- 1 cup spinach OR kale, packed

- 1 cup almond milk

5. Include organic food and food rich in fiber. Natural food choices ensure nutrients the body needs. Fibrous food provides energy by slowing digestion. You can have the best vigor throughout the whole day with food choices that are rich in fiber.

Some of the best energy providers are seen below.

- Chia seed yogurt

- Tempeh salad wraps

- Quinoa bowl

- Peanut butter banana

- Cranberry smoothie

To look alive throughout the day, you can make these plant-based dishes. Your friends and co-workers would be jealous of the energy you can maintain with these food picks. You will feel more productive and know you made the right meal plan choice.

This all boils down to knowing the facts that support that plant-based food choices are abundant in nutrients. Here is more information on a few of the nutrients that these food choices contain.

High Dietary Fiber

Manages body weight prevents constipation and reduces diabetes and heart disease risks. avocado (10.5 g/cup sliced serving), Asian pears (9.9 g/ medium-sized fruit), raspberry (8 g/cup), blackberry (7.6 g/cup), coconut (7.2 g/cup), figs (14.6 g/cup dried figs), artichokes (10.3 grams/ medium-sized piece), peas(8.6 g/cup cooked serving), okra (8.2 g/cup), acorn squash (9 g/cup baked serving), Brussels sprouts (7.6 g/cup), turnips (4.8 g/half a cup), black beans (12.2 g/cup), chickpeas (8 g/cup), lima beans (13.2 g/cup cooked serving), split peas (16.3 g/cup cooked serving), lentils (10.4 g/ cup cooked serving), almonds (0.6g/ six almonds or 1.9 g/ounce), flax seeds (3 g/ tablespoon), chia seeds (5.5 g/tablespoon, and quinoa (5 g/cup cooked serving).

Vitamin C

Sustains energy, fights diseases, reduces physical and emotional stress, and increases iron. Examples: peppers, particularly yellow bell peppers (95.4mg/10 strips or 52 grams), guavas (125.6mg/fruit or 376.7 mg/cup or 165 g), kale (80.4mg/cup), green kiwi (80.4mg/fruit or 166.9mg/cup sliced serving), broccoli (81.2mg/cup chopped serving), strawberries (10.6mg/large fruit or 10.6mg/cup sliced serving or 166 g), oranges (69.7mg/orange or 95.8mg/cup sections serving), cooked tomatoes (56.1mg/2 cooked tomatoes or 54.7mg/cup or 240 g), peas or mange tout (20.4mg/10 pods or 37.8mg/cup), and papaya (95.6mg/small fruit or 88.3mg/cup sliced serving).

Magnesium

Maintains healthy nerve and muscle function keeps the immune system healthy, maintains healthy heart rhythm, and builds strong muscles. Example: spinach (157mg/cup or 180 g), pumpkin and squash seeds (156mg/1 ounce handful or 28 g), lima beans (126mg/cup or 170 g), brown rice (86mg/cup or 195 g), almonds (79mg/1 ounce handful or 28 grams), dark chocolate – 85 percent cocoa (65mg/1 ounce square or 28 g), avocado (44 mg/1 cup cubed serving or 150 g), and bananas (32mg/1 medium fruit).

Potassium

Maintains electrolyte and fluid balance in the body. Examples: dried apricots (1511mg/ cup or 130 g), white beans (1004mg/ 1 cup or 170 g), avocado (975mg/1 medium fruit), potatoes (926mg/1 medium piece), acorn squash (896mg/cup or 205 g), spinach (839mg/cup or 180 g), white button mushrooms (555mg/cup or 156 g), and bananas (422/1 medium fruit).

Remember that the plant-based diet lacks in Vitamin B12. You can adequately accomplish your health goals by including nutritional yeasts in your meal plan. It also makes an excellent substitute for cheese.

Your body will always have the best feeling because plant-based food contains vital nutrients. You will see that you can perform better and achieve more since these nutrients support the body. Every day that you practice this healthy eating habit, you will have high energy and nutrients. You will stop worrying about "surviving" because you will enjoy living instead.

Develop the Right Diet Practices

The last small detail that helps achieve full health potential is proper development of plant-based diet practices, addressing the question: *How do you know you are on the right track with your dieting?* The answer is simple. You can differentiate this diet from other diets, and then adapt it according to your needs.

The following visual serves as a guide in comparing popular health diets.

Plant-Based	Vegan	Flexitarian	Reducetarian
-Prioritizes whole fruits, vegetables, and grains -Avoids or limits animal-based food and plant fragments	-Avoids animal products totally -Habits are based on ethical beliefs -Can still eat processed foods	-Eats mainly fruits, vegetables, and grains but allow meat and dairy products	-Chooses to eat less meat and dairy products

The plant-based diet stands out among the other diets because it provides allowances to animal-based food. You should consult your doctor with the best choices in adopting this healthy eating plan. Most professionals would suggest that this diet is a good food plan because of its health benefits.

Discovering the riches of the diet means you are uncovering the treasure of full health potential. Plant-based food gives strength and fitness to the body. It also provides plenty of energy and nutrients. You will be glad to eat more healthy choices to develop and enhance your health.

Key Takeaways

- The Plant-Based Diet is eating whole fruits and vegetables as well as avoiding or limiting eating animal-based food. It is also known as the Whole Food Plant-Based (WFPB) diet.

- The main food choices are whole fruits, vegetables, legumes, tubers, and whole grains.

- Animal-based food and plant fragments should be avoided or limited, making the diet unique compared to other popular diets.

- This diet provides a healthy and fit body by maintaining body weight, preventing diseases, and promising long life among other benefits.

- This diet also provides more energy and nutrients. Some of these sources are Chia seeds, fruit smoothies, raisins, and almonds.

Chapter 2: Implementing the Plant-Based Diet at Home

The first place where you can enjoy the riches of a healthy eating habit should be at home. You can start applying this food plan efficiently. The methods are not complicated and can even be considered "the fun highlights" of your daily routine. Here you will have a reliable guide towards implementing this food plan for your home and further maintain your nutrition goals.

Master the Grocery Basics

Sometimes you may find yourself stuck at the kitchen counter with a blank grocery list. You would not have to worry now since brainstorming ideas for your home's kitchen needs is simple with this excellent eating plan. The diet mainly keeps you imagining the best products from the fruits and vegetable section of the grocery. It will then make sure you would consider the right substitutes for animal-based and dairy products.

As you compose your grocery list at home, you can always refer to this guidebook and review the plant-based diet shopping list basics. The items are based on a 2,000-calorie plant-based plan.

Fruit Items

- Lemons. Lemon juice can help digestive problems and is best taken 30 minutes before eating.

- Grapefruit, blueberries, and limes are just a few examples of fruits low in sugar.

- Dried fruits are healthy additions to salads.

- In-season organic fruits should always be prioritized.

- Consider 2 cups of fruit intake daily.

Vegetable Items

- In-season organic vegetables are not only the most nutritious choices but also very affordable.

- Cruciferous vegetables are believed to be preventers of cancer.

- Cauliflower is a delightful cruciferous vegetable.

- Ensure 2 1/2 cups of vegetables daily.

Legumes

- Include lentils and beans when you need protein choices. There should be 5 1/2 ounces of protein daily intake for good health. Plant-based diet takers recommend having legumes daily.

Whole Grains

- Grains are "whole" when it has all three of

its components: the bran, germ, and endosperm parts.

- Faro is an excellent choice that offers magnesium, protein, and iron.

- Brown rice can be a 5-gram protein choice. It also provides calcium and potassium among other nutrients.

- About 6 ounces of whole grain daily intake is nutritious.

Substituting Dairy Products

- Drink almond milk since it is a low calorie and sugar option. It also contains fats good for the heart.

- Consider 4 grams of oat milk for protein. But this is high in calories and sugar.

- There are non-dairy milk products with Vitamin B12, which is indicated on nutrition labels.

- Include almond, soy, or coconut yogurts. Limit it to below 10 grams to avoid high blood sugar.

- About 3 cups of these milk and yogurt substitutes should be included in your food plan daily.

Your grocery list helps complete your food planning. The information on these plant-based items is relevant because they promise your home healthy meal options. You will be able to start maintaining a fit body beginning with your smart grocery list ideas.

Prepare Your Kitchen Kingdom

Before making a plant-based diet change, you should prepare your kitchen with the best equipment. You should invest in high-quality kitchen tools to ensure smooth cooking and eating experience. This section discusses different cooking approaches, and it is specific kitchen tools that will help deliver excellent plant-based preparation.

Pressure Cooking

- Electric cookers are recommendable since stove cooking can take up more time. Some electric cookers can also serve for slow cooking, rice cooking, and steaming.

- Pressure-cooking for this diet is mostly used for soups, frozen vegetables, and whole wheat like oatmeal.

- A 6-quart model is suitable for a family of 5 while 5-quart models are suitable for a household of fewer people.

Slicing and Chopping

- Pieces of 7-inch knives can be used for vegetables and big fruits like watermelon.

Bowls

- A large bowl would be great for salads, vegetables, and or bread. You should purchase a stainless one.

Blending

- Blenders would always be needed for your plant-based recipes. They are required for bean dips, smoothies, salad dressings, and puddings among others.

Food Processing

- Small food processors can mince or chop herbs.
- Food processors can help grate vegetables, smash beans, and slice.

With these kitchen tools, you can make scrumptious and nutritious plant-based meals. If these devices are in tip-top shape, you will enjoy cooking more. You would realize that the diet can also be a fun experience.

Create the Right Plant Based Adaptations

When you want to create your own plant based diet meal plan, you should consider adaptations that will adequately meet your nutrition needs. As mentioned in the previous chapter, this diet is not perfect. It lacks Vitamin B12 and some necessary fatty acids. Discover more advice on adaptations that will help achieve good health here.

Ensuring Vitamin B12

Again, Vitamin B12 is essential because it helps form blood cells and blood cell division. It also helps support the nervous system. Women who are breastfeeding need to be Vitamin B12 sufficient or the child would be at risk for apathetic, lethargic, and general survival. It is believed people should have 2 1/2 micrograms of vitamin B12 daily (Craig, W.J, PhD., MPH, RD 2015).

To ensure to get enough vitamin B12, including soy or rice milk in your food plan. Use nutritional yeasts that indicate vitamin B12 on their labels. You can also find cereals that are abundant with this nutrient.

Ensuring Necessary Fatty Acids

The plant-based diet may not provide enough omega-3 fatty acids. Remember, omega-3 fatty acids are recognized for fighting heart diseases. Likewise, you can include omega-3 fatty acids by cooking with soybean, flaxseed, or canola oil. You can also eat more walnuts.

Preventing Anemia

Some people believe that the plant-based diet lacks iron. But health experts and the clear food choices easily debunk this theory. Some plant-based food choices that provide lots of this mineral and prevent anemia are:

- Beans
- Turnip greens
- Kale
- Apricots
- Pastas

Ensuring Protein

Others believe that eating plant-based food means lack of protein. There is little evidence that this theory is correct. Many food choices offer protein. You should have protein-rich food picks in your food plans like baked beans, tofu, and medium-sized bagels.

Minimizing Meat

Nowadays, several beginner plant-based dieters join in on the global Meatless Monday campaign.

Similar initiatives can help you eat less meat and a more disciplined diet taker. You can cut the plates you have with meat to half of what you usually eat. Challenge yourself to go 10 days without chicken or other meaty favourites without cheating.

Note that you should progress in eliminating meat and other animal-based products at your own pace. You can also ask advice from your doctor. You will be making the calls about the right plant-based food adaptations with these pointers and ensuring your transition to a healthy diet would is smooth.

Nail the Keys to a Disciplined Diet

Got the big picture of a plant-based diet? Check.

Mcmorized the dos and don'ts of the healthy eating plan? Check.

Prepared your kitchen and jotted down necessary adaptations? Check.

These tasks are straightforward compared to facing

discipline-dieting anxieties, where the real challenge lies. You can overcome your worries with this reliable guide. Each step serves as a key that will unlock your abilities to achieving the best plant-based eating habits.

Step 1: There are no pressures.

Remember how you can start with Meatless Mondays? You should also keep reminding yourself there are no real pressures to be strict with this diet. You know in your mind and heart the main reasons why you made a healthy eating habit. You do not have to pressure yourself to achieve your nutrition goals right away. Just keep your motivations in mind and ease into transitioning.

You can begin with the Meatless Monday goal. Then the 10-day practice of eating specific meat. Then stretch the time to a month commitment. Avoid beating yourself up over failure or self-doubt and think about this key - No pressures!

Step 2: Aim for the mini-goals.

Write down the big goals of losing weight or becoming more fit on your vision boards at home and the office. Then include the mini-goals on your cell phone or laptop's Daily Tasks application. Mini-goals can be: Eat fish only ONCE this week and/or Take a dairy yogurt today, then forget it for the rest of the week.

The mini-goals will pave the way to success. If you tend to relapse, go back to the key of step 1 and remember there are no real pressures. Maintain in your daily things-to-do the central idea that: Mini-goals are achievable.

Step 3: Initiatives are the real actions.

The reality is that you can make all the plans in the world, but they will not count without real effort or actions. So, realize the mini-goals by keeping yourself "on the move." Ensure you check these accomplishments and not remain in inaction. The mini-goals and initiatives are the same. But the step of acting is higher than planning mini-goals because your actions become achievements when you finish them.

Some more examples of goals and initiatives to act upon are:

- Avoiding putting eggs on the grocery list, or dropping by the Dairy section.

- Cooking up all the eggs in your refrigerator or giving them to the neighbours.

- Eating no two-legged animals for two weeks.

- Cleaning out all animal-based products from the fridge

Therefore, handle the key of acting on initiatives with care.

Step 4: Find delight in the variety of plant-based food options.

With the practice of right adaptations, all plant-based recipes are healthy meals. Most of the ingredients are very affordable. There are many plates you can try cooking or ordering.

You also will never be bored because of the several food choices this diet offers. You can have more fun in making traditional recipes plant-based. You could make chicken burgers to black bean burgers. You can make a polenta pie or a pizza with caramelized onions and pesto.

The options are endless, and you would be motivated to maintain your diet. You would know that the key to finding delight in plant-based variety is essential to diet discipline.

Step 5: Room for a healthy break is available

To support the first step of having no pressure even further, you can make room for snacks or cheats. You can still make healthy eating choices with a break.

One way for a healthy break is making your weekend dedicated to "Step 4: Find delight in the variety of plant-based food options." Do a food experiment and make a no-animal meal applicable to the new diet. Have a fake meat on your plate, or try out one of this guide's recommended dairy substitutes. When you can make your "breaks" entirely plant-based, you are also finishing steps three and four. The mini-goals become big goals that are achievable too.

The key to making room for a healthy break makes the statement that you can relax and stay on your nutrition goals at the same time.

Step 6: Reinforce nutritious eating with other healthy practices.

Although the plant-based diet can give you access to a full health potential, you just cannot rely on nutritious eating habits alone. You must manage other healthy practices with the best diet. The most recommendable health practices are doing meditation or relaxing activities and incorporating exercise.

Meditation and relaxing activities like tai chi can

soothe your mind. You would be able to deal with a demanding boss or care for your busy family better if you have a calm mental state. You should take 5 minutes to shut out negative or bothersome thoughts to meditate instead. Prioritize fitting 10 minutes of quick yoga positions to release the body and mind tension. You will be glad you have these healthy practices in your schedule and belief that with the right eating habits, you are driven to do more.

Along the same lines, choosing to exercise two to three time a week can do wonders for your body's overall health. You can train each muscle group or body part once or twice a week. You can ask your doctor or personal trainer the best exercise practices for your full health potential. But you can begin immediately with non-gym exercises, like doing 3 sets of 10 squats is a good start, at home or hill sprinting for 20 yards at your neighbourhood park.

Small and short exercises prepare your body for the day. You will see when you exercise and eat right that you can perform more of theses exercises more confidently. Thus, the reinforcement of healthy practices should be a part of your everyday schedule and be a valuable part of your time.

Step 7: More review and education equates to more motivation.

Review this guide repeatedly to keep you disciplined. The more you read, the more you may discover and re-discover. Join plant-based diet groups on social media websites. Watch cooking videos and follow blogs about healthy dieting. You should be immersing yourself in this fantastic health world in order to encourage yourself to maintain your nutrition goals on a long-term basis. As you review and learn more, you will feel that your diet will bring you a lot of new opportunities, ideas, and connections. You will also impress your peers with all the health knowledge you have. In conclusion, discipline and continual education in the diet should be made into a thrilling practice.

Step 8: Go for a Plant-Based Diet with friends.

The last key to diet discipline is finding friends, loved ones, and support that can help your nutrition goals 100 percent. Tell them the reasons why the plant-based diet is beneficial for their health share or recommend this book to them. Then encourage them to join you in nailing the healthy eating habits together. It could serve as an excellent challenge that you and your loved ones could have together.

When you have someone to diet with you, you will be reminded to eat healthier, as well as monitor their well being too. There will be less pressure and you will have someone to confide to when you relapse and someone to remind you to stay on the journey. This person can be the "one friend you truly know" or someone you meet on social media groups. Most importantly, they should be someone that can be there to support you and vice-versa. The key to friendship inclusion with dieting practice is a fun and excellent concept to nail.

Nailing a disciplined food menu may feel and be hard. With these keys in mind, dedicate your time and effort to your diet and nutrition goals. You will be more confident in achieving rather than failing for the ultimate dream of full health potential.

Implementing a healthy eating habit at home involves more than knowing what to put in the kitchen or the keys to a disciplined diet. It entails you are ready to have a home that practices nutritious eating habits. The notes you have taken with this chapter will become very useful in creating a happy home environment and contribute to its improved health status.

Key Takeaways

- Implementing this diet at home ensures nutritious eating habits.
- On your grocery list you should prioritize:
    1. 2 cups of fruit daily
    2. 2 1/2 cups of vegetables daily
    3. 5 ounces of protein daily

4. 6 ounces of whole wheat daily

5. Vitamin B12 fortified products

6. Dairy substitutes like almond yogurt and or coconut milk

7. Items with omega-3 fatty acids like walnuts and canola oil

- Your kitchen should have high-quality appliances and gadgets that make plant-based recipes easy. These items should include a blender, sharp and heavy knives, an electric pressure cooker, bowls, and a food processor.

- A few of the right adaptations to the plant-based diet means ensuring you have enough protein and eliminating meat. Examples of protein choices are tofu and baked beans. You can remove meat at your own pace and with a realistic goal like a 10-day chicken-less food plan.

- Refer to the Keys of Nailing a Disciplined

Diet to maintain your nutrition goals. Some of the most important keys are: having no pressures, taking initiatives, reinforcing eating habits with other healthy practices, and dieting with friends among others.

Chapter 3: Becoming a Role Model of Nutrition

When you master the plant-based diet, you immediately become a role model of nutrition. Your peers and co-diet takers may expect that you know the fundamentals of good health. Your family should be able to see that you practice your diet at restaurants or cafes. The kids around you should be able to observe and mimic your nutritious eating habits. You also should know that some plant-based products can help you even avoid sicknesses and improve your image. This chapter is the best place to understand how to become an accurate model of nutrition with this diet.

Access the Advantages of Understanding Nutrition Facts

Plant-based diet takers usually make their food choices based on their knowledge about proper nutrition. The quality of health heavily relies on a person's eating habits; therefore, being able to remember the fundamentals of a healthy diet will always be a useful practice. Understanding the elements and concepts of nutrition facts are not complicated. They are also quick to review when making your grocery plans.

Body Mass Index

To determine if you are fit, you must know your Body Mass Index (BMI). The BMI identifies the body fat you carry based on your height and weight. It also can imply that you are at risk for any diseases. Your BMI validates obesity or underweight conditions and is categorized according to the following calculations:

Underweight – Below 18.5

Normal-18.5–24.9

Overweight- 25.0–29.9

Obesity- 30.0 and Above

Your doctor, nutritionist or personal trainer will be the best professional that can assist you to make the right plant-based adaptations to have a healthy BMI. You can also recall the suggestions in this book.

Calories

Calories are the body sources of energy. They work closely with carbohydrates, protein, and fat. They also create protein and amino acids through the body's metabolism. It should be noted the body burns calories to balance health. The body does need calories for energy, but too much calorie intake can lead to being overweight and ultimately, sicknesses. You should know your average calorie intake to fulfill your health needs. The right calorie amount is assessed by gender, age, and physical activity efforts.

It is recommendable to do your best in evaluating your physical activities. Physical activities are important considerations because it is what you use your energy for, and they also shape your fitness status. There are three types of physical activity:

1. Sedentary
2. Moderately active
3. Active

Sedentary activity is light physical activity or energy used to do simple daily tasks.

To be considered moderately active means you do activities that equate to walking 1.5 to 3 miles every day at 3 to 4 miles per hour, along with accomplishing simple daily tasks. To be active equates to 3 miles every day at 3 to 4 miles per hour, along with simple daily tasks. Zelman, MPH, RD, LD (2008) of WebMD determined the standard calorie intake for the public. Here are the guidelines for a daily diet:

Gender	Age	Sedentary	Moderately Active	Active

Female	19-30	2,000	2,000-2,200	2,400
	31-50+	1,800	2,000	2,200
Male	19-30	2,400	2,600-2,800	3,000
	31-50+	2,200	2,400-2,600	2,800-3,000

As you buy and make plant-based food, you can now check the nutrition fact labels and see if you meet your calorie intake needs.

Carbohydrates

Carbohydrates work with calories to provide energy. The United States Department of Agriculture (USDA) (2010) found that 45-65% of calories are credited to carbohydrates. Furthermore, carbohydrates break down into glucose, which is the body's primary energy source.

Partial grains and sugars create refined

carbohydrates. Refined carbohydrates are ill-advised for the body because they damage the body's health. But health experts stress that carbs are necessary for full health potential. Therefore, it is advised to avoid some sweets.

While a low carbohydrate diet can help an individual meet nutrition goals meant for weight loss, the plant-based eating plan allows you to consume the right carbohydrate and focus on whole grains, fruits, and vegetables. About 45-65 percent of calories equates to around 225-325 grams of carbs for a 2,000-calorie daily diet (Mayo Clinic Staff 2014).

Sugars

Sugars are a type of carbohydrates. They help provide energy and vitamin A through digestion. They add taste and texture to food. However, excessive amounts of sugar intake lead to illnesses.

Health professionals point out that sugars should

be viewed as carbohydrates. Carbohydrates should be more than half of the energy intake of the diet. Moreover, the American Heart Association suggests limiting the amount of added sugar to the following amounts:

- Men: 150 calories of the total amount of your daily calorie need about 9 teaspoons or 37.5 grams daily.

- Women: 100 calories of the total amount of your daily calorie need, about 6 teaspoons or 25 grams daily.

Furthermore, it is vital to distinguish between natural sugars, which are found in vegetables and fruits from added sugar, which are sugars added to foods, commonly regular table sugar. Added sugars are often indicated as high fructose corn syrup or sucrose in food labels. You should avoid added sugars as much as possible.

The natural sugars in vegetables and fruits, which are the focus of a plant-based diet, are perfectly fine. Aside from organic sugar, these healthy foods contain fiber, water, and various micronutrients.

Protein

This cell component is responsible for repairing and building of tissues in the body. Protein from plant and animal food sources is digested and broken down in the stomach to protein building blocks called amino acids. The human system then utilizes these amino acids to build and repair your body. Nine out of the 20 amino acids that your body needs, known as essential amino acids, is not synthesized by the body, so you must get them through food.

These 9 essential amino acids are:

1. Valine

2. Tryptophan

3. Threonine

4. Phenylalanine

5. Methionine

6. Lysine

7. Leucine

8. Isoleucine

9. Histidine

About 10-35 percent of your daily calorie intake should come from lean protein. Since you are limiting or avoiding animal-based protein in a plant-based diet, you can get them from these satisfying plant sources:

- Almonds
- Amaranth
- Artichokes
- Asparagus
- Black-eyed peas
- Black beans
- Broccoli
- Chia seeds
- Chickpeas

- Edamame
- Green beans
- Green peas
- Hemp milk
- Hemp seeds
- Lentils
- Nutritional yeast
- Oatmeal
- Peanut butter
- Pumpkin seeds
- Quinoa
- Soy milk
- Spinach
- Spirulina
- Tahini
- Tempeh

- Tofu

Fat

Similar to carbohydrates, fat has been demonized as fattening and unhealthy. But there is a distinctive difference between dietary fat and body fat.

Dietary fats are essential nutrients that provide the body with energy, helps protect the organs from damage, and boosts absorption of certain vitamins that are fat soluble, including vitamins D, A, K, and E.

You should avoid trans fat, which is the type of fat found in shortening, baked goods, and processed food. They are what is known as "bad fat," and they increase the risk of developing heart disease.

On the other hand, unsaturated fat or what is known as "good fat" help prevent heart disease and even help protect the heart. Nut butter, flaxseed, olive oil, avocados, and nuts are excellent sources of healthy fat in a plant-based diet.

Omega-3 fatty acids and other polyunsaturated fat are also essential for the body's proper functioning. However, unlike other fatty acids, the body cannot synthesize it. Walnuts, flax seeds, Chia seeds are only some of the best sources of plant-based omega-3 fatty acids.

About 20-35 percent of your daily intake should come from healthy dietary fat.

Vitamins

There are many different types of vitamins, and each one has its specific role and function in the body, and they are equally essential to maintain optimal health. Men and women have minute differences in the amounts of vitamins that the body needs specifically. However, in general, the body needs the following essential vitamins:

- Vitamin A
- Vitamin C

- Vitamin D
- Vitamin E
- Vitamin K
- B vitamins

A plant-based diet ensures you get your daily need of crucial vitamins since your meals are composed of plenty vegetables and minerals.

Minerals

Similar to vitamins, minerals are vital in maintaining the proper function of the body, each type has its specific role, and the body needs include the following:

- Sodium – maintains the fluid volume outside the cells and helps them function properly. Health experts suggest keeping your daily sodium intake to below 2,400 milligrams daily.

- Potassium – maintains the fluid outside and inside the cell, preventing the excessive rise of blood pressure when you intake high amounts of sodium. Tomatoes, potatoes, and bananas are rich sources of potassium.
- Calcium – helps build and maintain strong teeth and bones. Almond milk, and cheese are great sources of calcium.

However, since you are limiting or avoiding animal-based products, you can get your daily need of calcium from the following:

- Almond nut and butter
- Almonds
- Bok Choy
- Broccoli
- Chia seeds

- Dried figs
- Kale
- Kale
- Linseed
- Mustard greens
- Navy beans
- Okra
- Pak Choi
- Rice milk
- Soy milk
- Soy yogurt
- Soybeans
- Spring greens
- Tahini
- Tempeh
- Tofu

- Turnip greens

Other important minerals include iron, chloride, magnesium, phosphorus, and other trace minerals.

Water

Many of us overlook the importance of a properly hydrated body. Our body mass is made up of between 55-75 percent water. Even a few days without water can be harmful to your health. It is the core component of every cell in the body.

Water maintains the body's homeostasis, as well as transports nutrients to the cells, regulates the body temperature, aids in food digestion, and assists in removing waste products from the body.

- Adults should drink between 25 to 35 milliliters of fluid for every 1 kilogram of body weight, which totals to about 2-3 liters of fluid daily or 8 to 12 glasses of water.

If you are not getting enough fluid, you can suffer from fatigue, dizziness, dry skin, rapid heart rate, and even death.

Aside from drinking water, you can adequately hydrate your body by consuming foods with high water content, such as vegetables and fruits.

It would seem like it would take a great deal of effort to cram all these macronutrients and micronutrients into your diet. Luckily, it is more straightforward than it seems to get your daily nutrient intake. There is no need to follow any specific guide or list for a healthy diet meticulously unless you are on a restricted diet or you have a condition that entails you to develop a strict guideline. You only need to follow a diet in whole foods rich in whole grains, vegetables, and fruits. With a plant-based diet, you will be able to consume a hearty amount of all the essential nutrients you need with every meal. A healthy food menu is nutrient dense and can supply your body concentrated amounts of micronutrients with each serving.

Chapter 4: Begin the Day with Plant-Based Breakfasts

You ought to start each morning with a scrumptious and nutritious plant-based breakfast. These breakfasts provide you with the energy to do everything you need and begin the day with a superb feeling.

Oats to Love

Prep Time: *1* minute

Cook Time: *5* minutes

Serves: **2**

Ingredients:

- 1 cup rolled oats
- 1 cup of blueberries, frozen or fresh
- 1 3/4 cups of water
- 2 tablespoons of Chia seeds
- 2 cups almond milk, OR your milk of choice
- Agave nectar, to taste

Directions:

1. On a stovetop, boil the water in a pot.
2. Add the oats and continue boiling. Then put in the seeds.

3. Boil for 2-3 minutes. Lower the heat and stir when necessary.

4. Get two bowls. Put half a cup of blueberries in each of them. Pour the cooked oats over the fruits.

5. Stir the oats and then add the non-dairy milk. Add the agave to taste. Serve warm.

Calories:	**819** kcal
Total Carbohydrates:	**58.5** g
Sugar:	**15.6** g
Total Fat:	**64.6** g
Protein:	**14.4** g
Sodium:	**43** mg

Granola Energizer

Prep Time: **5** minutes

Cook Time: **20** minutes

Serves: **6**

Ingredients:

- 2 cups of oats
- 1 cup of nuts, should be raw and non-salted
- 1 cup of dried raisins
- 1 cup of dried flaked coconut
- 1/2 cup blanched almonds

- 1/2 cup of pepitas or pumpkin seeds

- 1/3 cup of maple syrup

- 1 teaspoon of cinnamon

- 1 teaspoon ginger powder

- 1 teaspoon garam masala

- 1 teaspoon coarse Celtic sea salt

Directions:

1. Preheat the oven to 350F.

2. Get some non-stick parchment paper and line a baking with it. Set aside.

3. In a large mixing bowl, put in the dried ingredients, nuts, and spices. Then stir and combine.

4. Put in the rest of the ingredients and stir well. You may use your hands.

5. Get the baking tray and spread the mixture evenly. Put it in the oven for 15 minutes.

6. Toss the granola, then spread it out again evenly. Bake it for another 10 minutes. It should come out brown.

7. Put in the raisins and flaked coconut. Stir gently to cool. More cooling will create a hard texture. Then it is practically ready to serve.

Calories:	**471** kcal
Total Carbohydrates:	**64** g
Sugar:	**29** g
Total Fat:	**20** g
Protein:	**10** g
Sodium:	**294** mg

The Pancake Solution

Prep Time: *5* minutes

Cook Time: *20* minutes

Serves: *4*

Ingredients:

- 1 cup of buckwheat flour
- 1 cup of almond milk, unsweetened
- 1 ripe banana, mashed
- 1 tablespoon ground flax
- 1 tablespoon of agave nectar

- 1 teaspoon of baking powder
- 1 teaspoon of baking soda
- 1/8 teaspoon of pink Himalayan salt
- Coconut oil
- Banana slices, raw honey, toasted almonds

Directions:

1. Get a large bowl. Put in the flour, baking powder and soda, ground flax, and salt. Mix the ingredients.

2. Put in the mashed banana, milk, and agave syrup. Mix them to dry the ingredients. The batter will turn out runny and thick.

3. Get a cast-iron skillet and grease it with the coconut oil. Heat it at over medium temperature.

4. Put 1/4 of the batter in the skillet and cook for 2 minutes. Small bubbles will appear. Flip the pancakes and cook again for 2 minutes.

5. Put on a plate and cover with a towel. This will keep it warm.

6. Repeat for more pancakes. Then top them with the banana slices, honey, and almonds.

Calories:	**465** kcal
Total Carbohydrates:	**65.2** g
Sugar:	**20** g
Total Fat:	**19.8** g
Protein:	**14.7** g
Sodium:	**437** mg

The Energy Porridge

Prep Time: **5** minutes

Cook Time: **25** minutes

Serves: **2**

Ingredients:

- 1/2 cup quinoa
- 1 cup oats
- 2 1/4 cups water
- 2 apples to be peeled, cored, and diced roughly
- 2 tablespoons coconut yogurt
- 1 tablespoons coconut chip or desiccated coconut
- 3 1/2 ounces fresh cherries
- A handful of fresh raspberries

- A pinch of mixed cinnamon, nutmeg, and ginger

- A pinch of extra cinnamon

- A pinch of extra freshly grated nutmeg

Directions:

1. In a pan, put in the quinoa, oats, and mixed spice. Add 2 cups of water. Boil it in low heat. Reduce to simmer, then cook for 10 minutes. Add water if necessary.

2. Make an apple compote by putting the apples in a pan. Cover it a ¼ cup of water, a pinch of cinnamon, and a pinch of nutmeg. Boil until it is tender. This should take 10 minutes. Drain and tip them into a food processor. To create smoothness, blitz them. Then put aside.

3. Divide the porridge into two bowls. Top them with a huge spoonful of apple compote. Add the other fruits and coconut

yogurt. Use the coconut chips as additional toppings. Serve warm.

Calories: **260** kcal
Total Carbohydrates: **51** g
Sugar: **17** g
Total Fat: **3** g
Protein: **11** g
Sodium: **55** mg

Start the Day with Salad

Prep Time: **20** minutes

Cook Time: **20** minutes

Serves: **4**

Ingredients:

For the salad:

- 1 pack of herb blend salad greens about 5 ounces
- 2 cups sliced strawberries
- 1/2 cup almonds, slivered
- 1/2 cups pepitas, salted and roasted
- 1/4 cup coconut bacon
- Coarse salt and black pepper for taste

For the coconut bacon:

- 1 1/2 cups unsweetened flaked coconut

- 1 tablespoon soy sauce
- 1 tablespoon pure maple syrup
- 1 1/2 teaspoons liquid smoke
- 1 1/2 teaspoons water
- 1/2 teaspoon smoked paprika
- 1/2 teaspoon fresh ground black pepper

For the black pepper vinaigrette:

- 3/4 teaspoon fresh ground black pepper
- 1/3 cup red wine vinegar
- 2/3 cup canola oil
- 1 teaspoon granulated sugar
- 1/2 teaspoon minced garlic
- 1/4 teaspoon salt

Directions:

1. Create the coconut bacon first by doing steps 2 to 4.

2. Preheat the oven to 325 F. Center the oven rack.

3. Whisk the soy sauce, syrup, liquid smoke, and water in a medium-sized bowl. Put in the coconut. Stir until the liquid is absorbed. On the top, sprinkle the paprika and black pepper. Stir to combine well.

4. Get a large rimmed baking sheet and line it with parchment paper. Spread the coconut flakes to create a layer. Make sure the flakes are spread evenly. Then bake until they are dark brown. This should take 10 minutes minimum.

5. Create the black vinaigrette next. Mix the ingredients (except the oil) in a small mixing bowl. Whisk them well. Slowly add a drizzle of canola oil, blending while you whisk.

6. Now finish the salad. Put the mix in a large bowl, and then sprinkle it with salt and black pepper. Toss for a good mixture. Put

in the strawberries, pepitas, almonds, and coconut bacon. Drizzle your servings with the dressing.

Notes: The bacon may burn easily. It should look crumbled.

Calories:	*591* kcal
Total Carbohydrates:	*14* g
Sugar:	*2* g
Total Fat:	*8* g
Protein:	*55* g
Sodium:	*145* mg

Rich Rice Pudding

Prep Time: *5* minutes

Cook Time: *10-15* minutes

Serves: *2*

Ingredients:

- 1 cup coconut milk (about 1/2 can)
- 1 cup cooked white or brown rice
- 1 tablespoon maple syrup or agave
- Dash cinnamon

Directions:

1. Pour the coconut milk in a small-sized pot and bring to a simmer over medium-high heat.
2. Add the maple syrup and stir to combine.
3. Add the rice and stir until the mixture is distributed evenly.

4. Simmer the mixture for 5 minutes or until the liquid is reduced and the mixture is thick.

5. Divide the mixture between 2 serving bowls. Sprinkle the top with cinnamon and serve.

Calories:	**640** kcal
Total Carbohydrates:	**87.4** g
Sugar:	**10.1** g
Total Fat:	**29.2** g
Protein:	**9.4** g
Sodium:	**24**mg

Merry to Eat Muffins

Prep Time: **5** minutes

Cook Time: **25-30** minutes

Serves: **12**

Ingredients:

- 3/4 cup soymilk
- 2 teaspoons baking powder
- 1/4 cup oil
- 1/2 cup sugar
- 1 teaspoon salt
- 1 cup frozen blueberries
- 1 1/2 cups flour

Directions:

1. Put the baking powder, flour, salt, and sugar in a mixing bowl and stir until well

combined.

2. Stir in the soy milk and the oil until well incorporated. Gently fold the blueberries into the batter mixture.

3. Line a 12-cup muffin pan with paper cups. Divide the batter between the muffin cups.

4. Bake in a preheated 400F oven for about 25 to 30 minutes or until the muffins are cooked through.

Calories:	***144*** kcal
Total Carbohydrates:	***23.4*** g
Sugar:	***10.2*** g
Total Fat:	***5*** g
Protein:	***2.2*** g
Sodium:	***203*** mg

Quick Quinoa for a Busy Day

Prep Time: *5* minutes

Cook Time: *15* minutes

Serves: *1-2*

Ingredients:

- 3/4 cups uncooked quinoa
- 3 walnuts, chopped
- 2 1/4 cups almond milk, divided
- 1 tablespoon maple syrup
- 1 tablespoon dried cranberries
- 1 tablespoon almond butter
- 1 persimmon, chopped

Directions:

1. Pour 2 cups of the almond milk in a saucepan and bring to a boil over high heat.

2. When the milk is boiling, add the quinoa and reduce the temperature to medium heat or the mixture to a simmer. Cover and simmer for about 15 minutes or the quinoa absorbs the milk.

3. Remove the saucepan from the heat. Pour in the remaining 1/4 cup almond milk and the almond butter. Stir until well distributed.

4. Transfer the mixture into serving bowl.

5. Add the rest of the ingredients. Serve and enjoy!

Calories:	*985* kcal
Total Carbohydrates:	*69.2* g
Sugar:	*15.5* g
Total Fat:	*76.3*g
Protein:	*18.4* g
Sodium:	*46* mg

A Delightful Chickpea Omelet Plate

Prep Time: *10* minutes

Cook Time: *20* minutes

Serves: *3 pieces* (6-inch each) omelets

Ingredients:

- 1 cup chickpea flour
- 1/2 teaspoon baking soda
- 1/2 teaspoon garlic powder
- 1/2 teaspoon onion powder
- 1/3 cup nutritional yeast
- 1/4 teaspoon black pepper
- 1/4 teaspoon white pepper
- 1 cup water
- 3 green onions (green and white parts), chopped

- 4 ounces mushrooms, sautéed, optional

Directions:

1. Put the chickpea flour, baking soda, nutritional yeast, black pepper, white pepper, garlic powder, and onion powder in a small-sized bowl and stir until well combined.

2. Pour the water in the flour mixture and stir until the mixture is a smooth batter.

3. Heat a frying pan over medium flame or heat. When the pan is hot, pour the batter into the pan, as if you are making a pancake. Sprinkle each omelet with 1-2 tablespoons of green onions, and if using, with sautéed mushrooms.

4. When the bottom of the omelets is browned, flip, and cook for 1 minute more or until cooked through.

5. Serve with spinach, salsa, tomatoes, hot sauce, or whatever plant-based topping you

want.

Calories:	**316** kcal
Total Carbohydrates:	**51** g
Sugar:	**7.7**g
Total Fat:	**5.1**g
Protein:	**21.5**g
Sodium:	**243**mg

Fabulous Fruit Tart

Prep Time: *2* hours, *30* minutes

Cook Time: *0* minutes

Serves: *6*

Ingredients:

For the crust:

- 2 cups raw walnuts, OR almond, pecan, or your preferred nut

- 7-12 Medjool dates, pitted (if not moist and sticky, soak in warm water for 10 minutes and drain

- 1/4 teaspoon sea salt, optional

For the filling:

- 1 1/2 cups mixed fresh fruit, divided (strawberries, blueberries, mango, kiwi, or your preferred fruits)

- 1/2 teaspoon vanilla extract

- 1/4 cup maple syrup, OR agave nectar

- 12 ounces firm silken tofu, patted dry and gently pressed in a clean towel for at least 15 minutes- 1 hour

- 2 tablespoons lemon juice, from 1 lemon

Directions:

1. Drain or press the tofu.

2. Meanwhile, prepare the crust. Put the walnut into a food processor. Pulse until processed until it resembles a semi-fine meal.

3. With the motor of the food processor running, add the dates 1 piece at a time through the spout until the mixture resembles a dough. The dough should hold its form when you squeeze them between 2 fingers. This will take about 7 to 12 dates, depending on their sizes.

4. Line a standard tart or pie pan, or a couple of 4 3/4-inch tart pans with parchment paper. Divide the crust dough between the pans, pressing into the pan to create uniform dough. You can put another parchment paper on top of the crust and then use a glass to even and press the crust in place firmly. Chill in the freezer until chilled.

5. Put the drained tofu, sweetener, vanilla, and lemon juice into a blender. Blend until the mixture is smooth and creamy, scraping the edges as needed.

6. When the crust is chilled, transfer the filling mixture in the crust. Chill for at least 2 hours, up to 4 hours.

7. When ready to serve, top with fruit and, if desired, serve topped with coconut whipped cream.

8. Store any leftovers in the refrigerator for up to a couple of days or freeze for long-term

storage.

Calories:	*375* kcal
Total Carbohydrates:	*27* g
Sugar:	*19* g
Total Fat:	*26* g
Protein:	*14.5* g
Sodium:	*119* mg

Chapter 5: Love Lunch Pack Solutions

Lunch can be said to be the most social meal of the day. You can show off your plant-based meals to your co-workers and friends. They would see that your nutritious eating habits are quite delightful to the eyes and taste buds as well.

The Most Desirable Chili Bowl

Prep Time: **10** minutes

Cook Time: **45** minutes

Serves: **6**

Ingredients:

- 1 red pepper, diced

- 3/4 cup dry red lentils, rinsed well in cold water then drained

- 1 3/4 cup water, plus more as needed

- 1 white or yellow onion, diced

- 1 jalapeño, diced with seeds

- 3 tablespoons tomato paste

- 4 cloves garlic

- 3 tablespoons chili powder, divided

- 2 tablespoons ground cumin, divided

- 2 tablespoons grapeseed or coconut oil

- 1 teaspoon smoked paprika

- 1/2 teaspoon each sea salt and black pepper, divided (have additional ones to taste)

- 2 cans (15-ounces) diced tomatoes (if unsalted, add more sea salt)

- 1 can (15-ounces) kidney beans, slightly

drained

- 1 can 15-ounces) black beans, slightly drained

- 1-2 tablespoons coconut sugar, OR maple syrup

- 1 can (15-ounce) corn, drained, optional

Directions:

1. Over medium flame or heat, heat a large pot. When hot, put in the oil, red pepper, and onion. Season with the salt and black pepper, then stir. Stir a lot for 4 minutes.

2. Get a pestle and mortar. Put in the jalapeno and garlic. Crush until it becomes a rough paste. Get the onion and red pepper, then put them in the large pot. Season with salt and black pepper again.

3. Put in 2 tablespoons of chili powder, 1 tablespoon of cumin, diced tomatoes, tomato paste, paprika, and water. Stir and mix well. Boil it low over medium flame or

heat.

4. When it boils, put in the lentils, and then reduce the heat medium-low, creating a gentle simmer. You should see bubbles, but there should be no more boiling occurring. Cook for 15 minutes, making the chili tender. Add water if it looks dry and if the lentils are not submerged.

5. Add the kidney and black beans, 1/4 of each salt and black pepper, and the rest of the cumin and chili powder. Stir to mix well.

6. Simmer over medium flame or heat, then reduce the heat low. Put in corn if you like. Cover then simmer gently for 20 minutes.

7. Add the seasonings for more taste.

Calories:	***320*** kcal
Total Carbohydrates:	***52.4*** g
Sugar:	***10*** g
Total Fat:	***6.8*** g

Protein: **15.9** g

Sodium: **427** mg

Plant-Based Meatloaf

Prep Time: **10** minutes

Cook Time: **55** minutes

Serves: **8**

Ingredients:

For the chickpea meatloaf:

- 2 cups panko breadcrumbs
- 2 celery stalks, chopped
- 2 carrots, diced
- 2 cans (14-ounce each), OR 3 1/3 cups cooked chickpeas, drained and rinsed
- 1/4 teaspoon black pepper
- 1/2 cup unflavored almond or soy milk
- 1 teaspoon liquid smoke
- 1 onion, diced

- 2 garlic cloves, minced
- 2 tablespoons ground flax seeds
- 2 tablespoons olive oil
- 2 tablespoons tamari or soy sauce
- 2 tablespoons tomato paste
- 3 tablespoons vegan Worcestershire sauce

For the maple glaze:

- 2 tablespoons maple syrup
- 2 tablespoons apple cider vinegar
- 1/4 cup tomato paste
- 1 teaspoon paprika
- 1 tablespoon soy sauce or tamari

Directions:

1. Preheat the oven to 375F. Lightly grease a 9-inch loaf pan with oil.

2. Working in batches as needed, put all of the meatloaf ingredients into a food processor.

Pulse until the chickpeas are broken and all the ingredients are mixed well, scraping the sides of the food processor as needed. DO NOT overblend. If working in batches, transfer the processed mixture in a large-sized mixing bowl and combine using clean hands.

3. Press the meatloaf mixture into the greased loaf pan. Bake in the preheated oven for 30 minutes.

4. While the meatloaf is baking, put all of the glaze ingredients into a small-sized bowl and stir until well combined.

5. After the 30 minutes are up, remove the meatloaf from the oven. Spoon glaze over the top of the meatloaf. Return to the oven and bake for about 20 to 25 minutes more.

6. Remove from the oven. Let cool for at least 10 minutes before slicing.

Notes: The longer the meatloaf sits, the firmer it

gets. If the meatloaf is soft to your liking, then let it sit for a couple minutes more. You can also make this a day ahead. Just reheat on serving day.

Calories: **580** kcal

Total Carbohydrates: **76.2** g

Sugar: **18.4** g

Total Fat: **15.6** g

Protein: **22.1** g

Sodium: **480** mg

Curried Potatoes in Thai Style

Prep Time: **15** minutes

Cook Time: **15-20** minutes

Serves: **4-5**

Ingredients:

- 1 can (14-ounce) coconut milk, regular
- 1 tablespoon oil
- 1/2 cup chopped cilantro and peanut mixture
- 1/2-1 cup broth or water
- 2 shallots, thinly sliced
- 2 sweet potatoes, peeled and cubed
- 2-3 tablespoons curry paste
- 3-4 cups fresh baby spinach
- Fish sauce, to taste

Directions:

1. If you are serving this over rice, which is highly recommended, then cook your rice before starting on the dish.

2. Put the oil in a nonstick pan and heat over medium-high heat. When the oil is hot, add the shallots and stir-fry until fragrant and soft.

3. Add the sweet potatoes and stir to coat with the oil. Add the curry paste and stir until well incorporated.

4. Add the broth and the coconut milk, stirring to combine. Simmer on low heat for about 10 to 15 minutes or until the dish is thick.

5. Stir in the spinach and cook until wilted.

6. Add half of the cilantro-peanut mixture, reserving the rest as topping.

7. Add a splash of fish sauce into the dish. Serve over cooked rice garnished with the remaining cilantro-peanut mixture.

Calories: **341** kcal

Total Carbohydrates: **21.6** g

Sugar: **4.9** g

Total Fat: **27.5** g

Protein: **7.8** g

Sodium: **63.6** mg

Perfect Pineapple Fried Rice

Prep Time: **10** minutes

Cook Time: **20** minutes

Serves: **4**

Ingredients:

- 1 1/2 cups pineapple, cut into 1-inch cubes, canned or fresh
- 1 1/2 tablespoons coconut oil
- 1 cup carrots, peeled and diced
- 1 cup green onion, chopped
- 1/2 cup red onion, diced
- 1/4 teaspoon red chili pepper flakes, optional
- 1-2 tablespoons tamari sauce, OR soy sauce
- 2 teaspoons fresh ginger, grated

- 2-3 garlic cloves, minced

- 3 cups cooked rice, preferably a day old

Directions:

1. Put the coconut oil in a large-sized wok or pan and heat on medium heat. When the oil is hot, add the ginger, garlic, onion, carrots, and chili pepper, and sauté for about 7 to 9 minutes or until the carrots are tender.

2. Add the pineapple pieces and sauté for about 4 to 5 minutes or until slightly browned.

3. Add the tamari, cooked rice, and green onions. Stir-fry and taste for flavor. Add a pinch of salt or ash of tamari as needed.

4. Stir-fry for about 4 to 5 minutes or until the rice is heated through and the ingredients are combined.

Notes: To make this dish more filling, add more veggies, beans, baked tofu, or toasted cashews. For the vegetable options, you can add mushrooms, zucchini, eggplant, green beans, peas, bok choy, broccoli, bell peppers, and more.

Calories:	**614** kcal
Total Carbohydrates:	**126.4** g
Sugar:	**8.9** g
Total Fat:	**6.2** g
Protein:	**11.5** g
Sodium:	**257** mg

A Valuable Vegetable Quiche

Prep Time: **15** minutes

Cook Time: **1** hour, **30** minutes

Serves: **8**

Ingredients:

For the crust

- 3 medium to large-sized potatoes (about 3 cups total when grated)
- 1/4 teaspoon of sea salt and black pepper
- 2 tablespoons olive oil, OR vegan butter

For the filling:

- 1 cup broccoli, chopped
- 12.3 ounces tofu, extra-firm silken, patted dry
- 3 tablespoons hummus

- 2 tablespoons nutritional yeast

- 3 garlic cloves, chopped

- 1 medium onion, diced

- 3/4 cup of cherry tomatoes, sliced into halves

- Sea salt and black pepper, to taste

Directions:

1. Preheat the oven to 450F. With nonstick cooking spray, lightly grease a 9 1/2-inch pie dish.

2. Grate 3 cups worth of potatoes. Put the grated potato in the greased pie pan and then drizzle with the olive oil. Season with 1/4 teaspoon salt and 1/4 teaspoon pepper. Toss to evenly coat and then spread and press in the pie pan, layering evenly.

3. Bake in the preheated oven for about 22 to 27 minutes, cooking until the crust is golden brown. Set aside.

4. While the crust is browning, prepare the garlic and vegetables and put into a baking pan. Toss to coat with a generous pinch pepper and salt and 2 tablespoons of olive oil. Put in the oven and cook along with the crust. When you remove the baked crust out from the oven, reduce the oven temperature to 400F and continue cooking the veggie mixture until golden brown and soft, about 20 to 30 minutes total. When the veggies are cooked, remove from the oven and set aside.

5. Reduce the oven temperature to 375F.

6. Put the drained tofu into your food processor. Add the hummus, nutritional yeast, 1/4 teaspoon salt, and 1/4 teaspoon black pepper, and process until well combined. Set aside.

7. Put the roasted vegetables into a large mixing bowl. Add the mixture of tofu and toss until coated. Transfer the veggie

mixture into the prepared crust, spreading the layer evenly.

8. Bake at 375F for about 30 to 40 minutes, cooking until the top is firm and golden brown. If you notice the crust is starting to get brown fast, tent the crust edges loosely with a piece of foil.

9. When the quiche is cooked, let cool for a couple of minutes. Serve with chopped green onion or fresh herbs.

Notes: Store leftovers in a loosely covered container and keep in the fridge for maximum of 2 days. When ready to serve, reheat in a 350F oven or in the microwave.

Calories:	*178* kcal
Total Carbohydrates:	*20.1* g
Sugar:	*2.8* g
Total Fat:	*8.7* g
Protein:	*7* g
Sodium:	*180* mg

Lasagna for my Lunchbox

Prep Time: *5* minutes

Cook Time: *1* hour and *30* minutes

Serves: *8-10*

Ingredients:

- 10 ounces gluten-free lasagna noodles
- 3 minced garlic cloves
- 2 big handfuls spinach
- 4 cups marinara sauce (32-ounces)
- 1 cup vegetable broth
- 3/4 cup of raw cashews, soaked overnight in water and drained
- 16 ounces of chopped mushrooms (use many types)
- 1 tablespoon coconut aminos, OR tamari

- 1 teaspoon of dried thyme

- To sauté, use coconut oil, vegetable broth, or grape seed.

- Optional: Nutritional yeast,

Directions:

1. Preheat your oven to a temperature of 350F.

2. In a large-sized skillet, put the oil, broth, or grape seed and heat over medium. Wait until the smell is produced. Put in the mushrooms, thyme, and tamari. Stir for 6 minutes. Wait for the broth to be created.

3. With a high-powered blender, mix the cashews and vegetable broth. You would want the texture to be smooth, for about 5 minutes. Put the heat on medium-low. Allow the mix to simmer, the sauce to thicken, and stir well. Add the spinach, then stir again for one more minute.

4. Make the lasagna after creating the sauce.

5. Get an 11x8-inch baking dish. Spread one-third of the sauce on its bottom. Put 1 layer of the noodles on the sauce. Cover it with 1/2 of your mushroom cream. Put another 1 layer of the noodles and 1/3 of the sauce to cover it. Put in the rest of the mushroom cream. Make one layer more of the noodles and then cover with the rest of the sauce.

6. With an aluminum foil, cover the lasagna, and then bake for half an hour. Take off the foil. You may add nutritional oil and then bake for 15 minutes. Allow the dish cool before serving, about 5 minutes.

Calories: *350* kcal

Total Carbohydrates: *27* g

Sugar: *3* g

Total Fat: *17* g

Protein: *23* g

Sodium: *570* mg

A Triple-B Burger

Prep Time: *5* minutes

Cook Time: *1* hour and *10* minutes

Serves: *3*

Ingredients:

- 1 pack of tempeh (8-ounces)
- 1 tablespoon of olive oil
- 1 cup of finely chopped yellow onion
- 1 cup of lightly toasted walnuts
- 1/2 cup all-purpose flour
- 2 minced cloves garlic
- 1 can lentils, drained and rinsed (15-ounces)
- 3 tablespoons of vegetable oil
- 1 teaspoon dried basil
- 1 teaspoon sea salt

- 1 pinch of freshly ground black pepper

Directions:

1. Steam out the tempeh for 20 minutes to remove bitterness.

2. Cut the tempeh into 6 small portions. Put it in the basket for a steam. Cook for another 20 minutes.

3. In a sauté pan of medium size, heat the olive oil over medium-high. Put in the onions, and then sauté lightly. They should look a little brownish.

4. Put in the garlic and cook for one minute. Put it in a big casserole for cooling.

5. Put the cooled garlic and onion in a food processor. Put in the tempeh, walnuts, dried basil, lentils, flour, salt and black pepper. Slowly pulse it. The nuts will break and create the vegetable burger mix.

6. Mix the ingredients in a bowl with your hands. Taste the mixture and add more salt

and black pepper if necessary.

7. Cut out patties from the mixture 4 oz. in size. In between 2 sandwich bags, press down the patties. Shape the patties round or in any form.

8. Put them in the refrigerator overnight.

9. Heat the vegetable oil over medium-high. Cook 3 patties for 4 minutes each side.

10. Top with red onion, tomato, and lettuce. Serve.

Calories:	**454** kcal
Total Carbohydrates:	**22** g
Sugar:	**7** g
Total Fat:	**22** g
Protein:	**25** g
Sodium:	**1,175** mg

An Enchanting Enchilada Dish

Prep Time: *15* minutes

Cook Time: *5* minutes

Serves: *4*

Ingredients:

- 1 medium avocado
- 1/2 cup black beans, canned
- 1/2 cup chopped carrot
- 1/2 cup cilantro
- 1/2 cup corn, canned
- 1/2 cup edamame, shelled
- 1/2 cup green enchilada sauce
- 1/2 cup red bell pepper
- 1/2 cup red tomato, chopped or sliced
- 1/2 cup white mushrooms, slices or pieces

- 2 cloves garlic

- 2 stalks green onion

- 6 medium corn tortillas

Directions:

1. Put the carrots, mushrooms, green onions, and garlic into a food processor and pulse until combined and the mixture is slightly chunky.

2. Grease a frying pan with oil. Put the carrot mixture in the pan. Add the tomato, black beans, corn, edamame, and bell pepper, and sauté until cooked and heated thoroughly.

3. Arrange the corn tortillas on a baking sheet. Divide the carrot mixture between the corn tortillas. Drizzle with green enchilada sauce and top with vegan cheese.

4. Bake in a preheated 375F oven for about 5 minutes or until the vegan cheese is melted.

5. Top with avocado slices and cilantro. Serve

while still warm.

Notes: For a classic version, divide the carrot mixture into whole-wheat tortillas, roll up, and put in a baking dish. Drizzle with enchilada sauce and top with the vegan cheese. Bake in a preheated 375F oven for about 5 to 7 minutes or until the vegan cheese is melted. Top with avocado slices and cilantro. Serve while still warm.

Calories:	*555* kcal
Total Carbohydrates:	*48.2* g
Sugar:	*4.1* g
Total Fat:	*36.1* g
Protein:	*13.8* g
Sodium:	*238* mg

Tasty Tofu

Prep Time: **15** minutes

Cook Time: **15** minutes

Serves: **4**

Ingredients:

- 1 pound tofu, firm or extra firm, drained and pressed
- 1/2 cup cooked quinoa
- Bottle of your favorite healthy, thick BBQ sauce, OR your preferred sauce

Directions:

1. Preheat the oven to 425F.
2. Line a baking sheet with a silicone mat or a parchment paper. Put a wire on top of the mat or paper.
3. Slice the pressed tofu into chicken nugget

size pieces, about 1/4-inch thick each. Working with 1 piece at a time, dip the tofu nuggets in the BBQ sauce and generously coat with the cooked quinoa. Put the coated tofu nuggets on the wire rack. Continue until all the tofu pieces are coated. This step can get a bit messy and you may want to pat some extra quinoa to coat each piece.

4. Cook in the preheated oven for about 15 to 20 minutes, or until the quinoa coating is crispy and browned.

5. Serve with BBQ sauce if desired.

Calories: **181** kcal

Total Carbohydrates: **38.6** g

Sugar: **16.9** g

Total Fat: **8.1** g

Protein: **14.2** g

Sodium: **710** mg

A Vegetable Wrap Wonder

Prep Time: **20** minutes

Cook Time: **0** minutes

Serves: **2** wraps

Ingredients:

- 4 large-sized collard leaves
- 2-3 ounces alfalfa sprouts
- 1/2 teaspoon ginger, grated
- 1/2 teaspoon garlic, minced
- 1/2 lime
- 1 teaspoon extra-virgin olive oil
- 1 tablespoon tamari, OR coconut aminos
- 1 red bell pepper
- 1 cup raw pecans
- 1 avocado

Directions:

1. Wash the collard leaves. Cut off the stems at the bottom of the leaves, the portion that has no leaves on them. Put the leaves in a mixture of warm water and juice of 1/2 a lemon. Let soak for 10 minutes. When the 10 minutes are up, dry the leaves using paper towels. With a knife, thinly slice down the central stems to make the leaves easier to bend later for wrapping.

2. Slice the pepper and the avocado.

3. Put the pecans in a food processor. Add the olive oil, garlic, ginger, and tamari. Pulse until the ingredients is combined and clump together.

4. Into each collard leaf, layer the nut mixture, avocado slices, and red pepper slices. Drizzle with lime juice and then top with the alfalfa sprouts. Fold the leaf over the bottom and the top, and then wrap the sides up. Slice each collard wrap into halves. Serve.

Calories: **666** kcal

Total Carbohydrates: **25.1** g

Sugar: **6.1** g

Total Fat: **60.4** g

Protein: **6.1** g

Sodium: **514** mg

Chapter 6: Dig in with Plant Based Dinners

When the day is over, it's great to wind down and relax with hearty and filling pant-based dinners recipes. Here are 10 dishes that will complete your day.

Vietnamese Noodles for the Soul

Prep Time: **15** minutes

Cook Time: **35-40** minutes

Serves: **4**

Ingredients:

- 1 large onion, peeled and quartered
- 1 star anise
- 1 tablespoon coconut aminos
- 1-inch piece of ginger, peeled and sliced in half

- 2 cinnamon sticks
- 2 garlic cloves, smashed
- 2 tablespoons fish sauce
- 3 large-sized zucchini
- 3 whole cloves
- 4 large-sized eggs
- 8 cups vegetable broth
- Salt to taste

For topping:

- 1 cup bean sprouts
- 1-2 limes, sliced
- 2 green onions, chopped
- Cilantro
- Mint leaves
- Red pepper flakes

Directions:

1. With the cut side facing down, put the ginger and the onion in a skillet set over medium-high heat. Cook the ginger for about 3-4 minutes and the onion for about 5 minutes, turning them halfway through the cooking time. Transfer the cooked onion and ginger into a stockpot.

2. Put the cinnamon stick, star anise, garlic, and clove in the skillet. Stir for about 30 seconds over medium-high heat or until the spices are fragrant. Turn the heat off. Transfer the spices to the stockpot.

3. Add the vegetable broth into the pot and bring to a boil. When the broth is boiling, reduce the heat to a simmer. Add the coconut aminos, fish sauce, and about 1 tablespoon salt, and simmer covered for about 30 minutes. There should not be any bubbles bubbling.

4. While the broth is simmering, wash the

zucchinis clean and then chop the ends off. Using the C-blade of a spiralizer, spiralize the zucchini into noodles. If you do not have a spiralizer, use a vegetable peeler to peel along the sides of the zucchini, making fettuccine-like pieces. You can also use a knife to carve strips on the zucchini until you reach the core and then slice the zucchini into long, thin pieces. Cut the zucchini noodles into shorter pieces using kitchen scissors if desired to make them more manageable.

5. Divide the noodles between 3-4 bowls.

6. When the broth is ready, strain the spices and return the broth to the pot. Taste the broth and add more salt as needed.

7. Fill each bowl with zucchini noodles with broth. Top with cilantro, mint, bean sprouts, lime, and red pepper flakes. Squirt about 1 tablespoon lime juice into the noodles.

Calories:	**252** kcal
Total Carbohydrates:	**24.6** g
Sugar:	**8.5** g
Total Fat:	**9** g
Protein:	**22.5** g
Sodium:	**2369** mg

Effortlessly Made Pizza

Prep Time: *5* minutes

Cook Time: *25* minutes

Serves: *4*

Ingredients:

- 1 cup water
- 1 tablespoon olive oil
- 1/2 cup marinara, OR pizza sauce
- 1/2 cup vegan mozzarella cheese
- 2 cups chickpea flour
- 2 teaspoons olive oil
- Dash salt
- Handful shredded kale

Directions:

1. Preheat the oven to 375F. Line a baking pan with parchment paper.

2. Put the flour in a medium-sized bowl. Add the water, salt, and 2 teaspoons olive oil and stir until mixed thoroughly.

3. Spread the dough into 1 large 1/4-inch thick pizza crust shape or 4 small 1/4-inch thick pizza crusts. Place the crust in the prepared baking pan.

4. Bake in the preheated oven for about 15 to 20 minutes or until the edges are slightly crisp.

5. While the crust is baking, toss the kale with 1 tablespoon olive oil.

6. When the crust is cooked, remove from the oven. Flip the parchment paper and crust upside down on the baking sheet. Gently pull the baking sheet away from the crust.

7. Spread the sauce over the crust. Layer the

kale on the sauce and then sprinkle with vegan cheese.

8. Bake in the oven for about 5 to 7 minutes. Slice and enjoy!

Calories:	**480** kcal
Total Carbohydrates:	**67.8** g
Sugar:	**13.5** g
Total Fat:	**15.2** g
Protein:	**21.1** g
Sodium:	**256** mg

Cobbler Crave Creator

Prep Time: *10* minutes

Cook Time: *45* minutes

Serves: *6*

Ingredients:

- 1 cup rolled oats
- 1/2 cup roughly chopped pecans
- 1/4 cup all-purpose flour, OR additional 1/4 cup almond meal
- 1/4 cup almond meal
- 2 packed light tablespoons muscovado sugar, OR brown sugar
- 2 tablespoons coconut sugar, OR more brown sugar
- 4 tablespoons olive oil, OR coconut oil, PLUS more for coating the pan

- 7-8 pieces ripe peaches, halved, pitted, and chopped

- A couple of cherries, pitted, chopped

- Pinch sea salt

Directions:

1. Preheat the oven to 350F. Lightly grease a square 8-inch baking dish with the olive oil.

2. Put the chopped fruit in the dish as you chop them and then spread them in an even layer in the dish.

3. Put the rest of the ingredients in a mixing bowl, including 4 tablespoons of olive oil. Using a wooden spoon or clean hands, mix until well combined.

4. Put the crumble mixture on top of the fruit layer, spreading in an even layer.

5. Bake in the preheated oven for about 40 to 45 minutes or until the top is golden and crisp and the fruit is bubbling.

6. Serve as is or with your favorite plant-based ice cream.

7. Store any leftovers in the fridge for up to 2 to 3 days.

Calories:	*288* kcal
Total Carbohydrates:	*33* g
Sugar:	*17* g
Total Fat:	*16.7* g
Protein:	*5* g
Sodium:	*3* mg

Plant-Based Casserole

Prep Time: **20** minutes

Cook Time: **1** hour, **15** minutes

Serves: **4-6**

Ingredients:

- 10 ounces super firm or extra-firm organic tofu, cubed

- 12 ounces mixture of baby carrots, snow peas, and broccoli florets, OR 1 bag (12-ounce) stir-fry vegetables

- 3 cups cooked rice, OR cooked cauliflower rice or quinoa

- 8 ounces tempeh, cubed

For the teriyaki sauce:

- 1/2 teaspoon garlic powder, OR 1 garlic clove, minced

- 1/2 teaspoon ground ginger, OR 1 teaspoon freshly grated

- 1/4 cup pure maple syrup, OR pure cane sugar or coconut sugar

- 2 tablespoons cornstarch, OR 3 tablespoons tapioca flour PLUS equal amount of water

- 3/4 cup tamari, OR coconut aminos, or low-sodium soy sauce

- 3/4 cup water

Directions:

1. Preheat the oven to 400F.

2. Drain the tofu and put between a folded clean towel. Put a heavy pot on top of the towel to squeeze out excess liquid for 10 minutes. You can skip this step if you are using super firm tofu.

3. Once the tofu is squeezed out, slice into 3/4 to 1-inch cubes. Slice the tempeh into 3/4 to 1-inch cubes as well.

4. Put the garlic, ginger, maple syrup, water, and tamari into a small-sized saucepan. Stir to combine and bring the mixture to a boil. When the mixture is boiling, reduce the heat to low and cook for 1 minute. Add 1-2 tablespoons more of maple syrup if you want a sweeter sauce.

5. Put the cornstarch and water into a small-sized bowl and mix until the mixture is smooth. Pour the cornstarch slurry into the saucepan and cook for about 1 minute or until the sauce is thick. Remove the saucepan from the heat and set aside.

6. Put the tempeh and the tofu into a medium-sized bowl. Add about 3/4 cup of the teriyaki sauce and toss gently to coat.

7. Line a baking sheet with Silpat or parchment paper. Spread the tempeh and tofu on the baking sheet, spreading them evenly. Put the baking sheet in the middle rack of the oven and bake for 40 minutes.

8. When the 40 minutes are up, reduce the oven temperature to 350F.

9. Cook the rice following the package directions.

10. Steam the vegetables in a bamboo steamer or whatever method you prefer.

11. Put the cooked rice, steamed vegetables, and baked tempeh-tofu in a casserole dish. Add more teriyaki sauce, leaving a small amount of the sauce for serving. Toss until the ingredients are well coated with the teriyaki sauce.

12. Put the dish in the oven and bake for about 10 to 15 minutes or until heated through.

13. Divide the casserole between 4 to 6 serving bowls. Drizzling each serving with the reserved sauce.

Notes: If you can't find tempeh, then use 1 whole block (14-ounces) of tofu instead. If you'd like to use only tempeh for your casserole, then use 2 packages (8-ounces each). You can also replace one of the vegetable ingredients with red bell pepper or spring peas or any vegetable that you prefer.

Calories:	***839*** kcal
Total Carbohydrates:	***146.1*** g
Sugar:	***12.9*** g
Total Fat:	***11.8*** g
Protein:	***36.4*** g
Sodium:	***3222*** mg

A Surprising Stew

Prep Time: **15** minutes

Cook Time: **30** minutes

Serves: **8** cups

Ingredients:

- 1 1/2 cups chickpeas, cooked
- 1 cup brown lentils, soaked for a couple of hours beforehand
- 1 cup carrot coins
- 28 fluid ounces canned diced tomatoes
- 2 teaspoons extra-virgin olive oil
- 2 medium garlic cloves, minced
- 2 cups zucchini, diced
- 2 cups water
- 2 cups loosely packed kale, de-stemmed

- 1/2 white onion

- 1 teaspoon parsley

- 1 teaspoon oregano

- 1 teaspoon dried basil

- 1 tablespoon fresh sage, minced

- Salt and black pepper, to taste

Directions:

1. Put the olive oil in a pan and heat over medium flame or heat for about 1 minute. Add the onion, garlic, and carrots, and sauté for about 2 minutes or until the onions start to become translucent.

2. Add the chickpeas, zucchini, tomatoes, lentils, dried herbs, and water. Stir until well combined and bring to a boil. When the mixture is boiling, cover the pot and simmer for 20 minutes.

3. When the 20 minutes are up, remove the pot from the heat and remove the lid. Stir in

the kale and sage.

4. Cover again with the lid and let the kale cook for about 5 to 10 minutes in the residual heat until wilted.

5. Season to taste with salt and black pepper.

Notes: If using uncooked chickpeas, soak them overnight in water, rinse, and cook in a separate pot for about 30 minutes before cooking the stew.

Calories:	***259*** kcal
Total Carbohydrates:	***44.5*** g
Sugar:	***8.6*** g
Total Fat:	***3.7*** g
Protein:	***14.6*** g
Sodium:	***42*** mg

A Tempeh Treat

Prep Time: **35** minutes

Cook Time: **10-20** minutes

Serves: **4-6**

Ingredients:

- 1 avocado, peeled, pitted, and sliced
- 1 cup microgreens
- 1 pound tempeh, cut into square patties
- 1 tablespoon olive oil, extra-virgin
- 1 yellow onion, peeled, halved, and sliced
- 1/3 cup BBQ sauce

Directions:

1. Put the tempeh patties in a shallow dish. Pour the BBQ sauce over the patties, covering them and then turning the patties to coat each side well with the sauce. Set aside.

2. Coat the bottom of a sauté pan with olive oil and heat over medium flame or heat. When the oil is hot, add the onion and sauté for about 30 minutes or until caramelized. Remove from the heat and set aside.

3. Grease a grill with cooking spray and then heat to medium-high. Alternatively, you can preheat the oven to 400F.

4. Remove the tempeh from the dish and put on the grill or bake in the oven right in the shallow dish.

5. If grilling, cook for about 10 minutes or until dark grill marks appear on the patties, turning them once during the cooking time.

6. If baking, cook for 20 minutes, turning the patties once.

7. Place the grilled or baked tempeh on serving plates. Place slices of avocado on top of the tempeh patties. Top with the microgreens and the caramelized onions.

8. Serve with more BBQ sauce as desired. Enjoy!

Calories:	**394** kcal
Total Carbohydrates:	**25.2** g
Sugar:	**6.9** g
Total Fat:	**25.7** g
Protein:	**22.3** g
Sodium:	**248** mg

Oh My! Bulgur Pilaf!

Prep Time: **10** minutes

Cook Time: **30** minutes

Serves: **2**

Ingredients:

- 1 tablespoon garlic, finely chopped
- 1 cup bulgur
- 1/2 teaspoon salt
- 1/3 cup pitted dates, chopped
- 12 cups mustard greens, thinly sliced, (around 1 bunch), remove the tough stems
- 2 shallots, chopped
- 2 tablespoons chopped walnuts
- 2-3 tablespoons of water
- 6 teaspoons walnut oil, OR extra-virgin

olive oil, divided

- 4 teaspoons of white-wine vinegar

Directions:

1. Prepare the bulgur following the package instructions. Transfer to a colander, rinse under running cool water and drain.

2. Toast the walnuts in a small-sized dry skillet on medium-low heat for about 2 to 3 minutes or until fragrant and lightly browned, stirring frequently. Remove from heat and set aside.

3. Put 5 teaspoons walnut oil into a large-sized skillet and heat on medium-low flame or heat. When the oil is hot, add the shallots and sauté for about 4-6 minutes or until they begin to brown. Add the garlic and sauté, frequently stirring, for around 15 seconds or until fragrant.

4. Add the dates, mustard greens, and 2 tablespoons of water. Cook for about 4

minutes or until the water evaporates and the mustard greens are soft, occasionally stirring. Add 1 tablespoon of water if the skillet becomes dry before your mustard greens are tender. Add the vinegar and salt. Add the bulgur and stir for about 1 minute or until thoroughly heated.

5. Drizzle the 1 teaspoon of walnut oil and then sprinkle the toasted walnuts over the dish. Serve.

Calories:	*196* kcal
Total Carbohydrates:	*31* g
Sugar:	7 g
Total Fat:	7 g
Protein:	7 g
Sodium:	*222* mg

Sweet Potatoes and Kale from Africa

Prep Time: **15** minutes

Cook Time: **55** minutes

Serves: **6**

Ingredients:

- 3-4 small sweet potatoes
- 1/4 cup pine nuts
- 1 cup wild rice
- 1 bunch kale
- Chili powder
- Cumin
- Ground mustard
- Salt and black pepper, to taste

Directions:

1. Slice the sweet potatoes into cubes and put into a parchment paper-lined baking dish. Toss and lightly coat with olive oil. Spread the sweet potato cubes evenly in the baking dish.

2. Bake in a 400F preheated oven for about 30 to 40 minutes or until fork tender.

3. Meanwhile, cook the wild rice according to the package directions.

4. When both the sweet potato cubes and rice are cooked, toast the pine nuts in a skillet over medium flame or heat for about 5 to 10 minutes.

5. Chop the kale into rough pieces.

6. Put the rice, sweet potato cubes, kale, and pine nuts in a large mixing bowl. Toss to incorporate and then season with the spices to taste.

7. Serve while still warm. Enjoy!

Calories:	**234** kcal
Total Carbohydrates:	**45** g
Sugar:	**5.5** g
Total Fat:	**4.2** g
Protein:	**6.7** g
Sodium:	**42** mg

A Nutritious Pasta Plate

Prep Time: *5* minutes

Cook Time: *25* minutes

Serves: *3*

Ingredients:

For the roasted chickpeas:

- 1 can chickpeas
- 1 tablespoon extra-virgin olive oil
- 1/2 teaspoon garlic powder
- Salt and black pepper, to taste

For vegetable noodles:

- 2 zucchinis
- 2 tablespoons of your favorite pesto
- 1 teaspoon garlic, minced
- 1 tablespoons extra-virgin olive oil

- 1 tablespoon water

- 1 medium-sized sweet potato, OR 1/2 large-sized sweet potato

Directions:

1. Preheat the oven to 425F.

2. Drain and rinse the chickpeas and, if desired, pick off any skins. Put rinsed chickpeas into a bowl. Add the seasonings and the olive oil. Toss to coat evenly. Spread the chickpeas on a baking sheet and roast in the preheated oven for 25 minutes, flipping the peas halfway through the cooking time.

3. While the chickpeas are roasting. Spiralize the zucchini and the potato into noodles using the C-blade of a spiralizer. If you do not have a spiralizer, use a vegetable peeler to peel along the sides of the zucchini and potato, making fettuccine-like pieces. You can also use a knife to carve strips on the zucchini until you reach the core and then

slice the zucchini into long, thin pieces. Put the zucchini noodles into separate bowls.

4. When there are only 10 minutes left of the chickpea roasting time, put a skillet on the stovetop an heat over medium flame or heat. When the skillet is hot, add the olive oil, garlic, water, and the sweet potato noodles. Cover the skillet and cook for about 5 minutes, stirring the noodles a few times.

5. Add the zucchini noodles, mix to combine and cook for 3 minutes. Remove the pan from the heat. Stir in the pesto until evenly coated.

6. Divide the vegetable noodles between 3 serving bowls. Divide the roasted chickpeas between the bowls, topping them on the vegetable noodles.

Calories:	***367*** kcal
Total Carbohydrates:	***47*** g
Sugar:	***10*** g
Total Fat:	***17*** g
Protein:	***10*** g
Sodium:	***435*** g

The Best Brown Rice Sushi

Prep Time: **30** minutes

Cook Time: **25** minutes

Serves: **3-4**

Ingredients:

For the sushi:

- 1 cup alfalfa sprouts
- 1 cup thinly sliced carrots
- 1 cup thinly sliced cucumber
- 1 red bell pepper, roasted or fresh, sliced,
- 4 sheets nori (dried seaweed)

For the rice:

- 1 2/3 cups water
- 1 cup short-grain brown rice, rinsed
- 1/2 teaspoon sea salt

- 2 tablespoons cane sugar, organic

- 3 tablespoons of rice wine vinegar

For serving (optional):

- Pickled ginger

- Sesame seeds

- Tamari, OR soy sauce

- Wasabi

Directions:

1. Pour the water into a medium-sized saucepan and boil. When the water is boiling, add the brown rice, stir to distribute, and reduce the flame to low heat. Cover the saucepan and simmer for about 18 to 25 minutes, or until the rice completely absorbs the water and tender. Drain off any excess water as needed.

2. While the rice is cooking, put the salt, sugar, and vinegar into a small-sized saucepan. Heat on medium heat, occasionally stirring

until the salt and sugar are dissolved. Put in a dish or a jar and refrigerate to cool until the rice is cooked.

3. When the brown rice is cooked, turn the heat off. Add the refrigerated vinegar and using a rubber fork or spatula, stir to incorporate, making sure not to overmix. The mixture will be wet at first, but the mixture will dry as the heat is released while you are stirring. Once the mixture is completely dry and sticky, then it's ready.

4. While the rice is finishing cooking, prepare the vegetables by slicing them into very thin pieces. You will not be able to roll the sushi if your veggies are too bulky.

5. Put a nori sheet on a sushi mat. Dip your hands in water. Pat a very thin cover of rice on the nori sheet, making sure that the layer is not too thick or you will not be able to roll the sushi. Leave about 1/2 an inch on top of the nori without rice.

6. At the 3/4 bottom of the rice layer, arrange the vegetables or your preferred layer in a lengthwise manner across the rice.

7. Staring at the side with the filling and using your fingertips, roll the nori with rice. Once the filling is covered with the nori and rice, hold the mat and roll it over the mold to compress it. Continue rolling and until the sushi is rolled completely. Repeat until all the rice and fillings are used, making about 5 to 6 rolls. Slice each roll into 6 equal pieces.

8. Serve right away with the wasabi, pickled ginger, tamari, and pickled ginger.

9. This dish is best when freshly made, but you can store leftovers in a container with a cover and keep refrigerated for up to 2 days.

Calories:	***438*** kcal
Total Carbohydrates:	***60.3*** g
Sugar:	***8.4*** g
Total Fat:	***1.9*** g
Protein:	***7.5*** g
Sodium:	***353*** mg

Chapter 7: Sweet Find Snacks

When you need something to perk you up in the middle of the day, these delicious plant-based snacks will surely energize you.

Burrito Bites

Prep Time: **15** minutes

Cook Time: **5** minutes

Serves: **6**

Ingredients:

- 1 1/2 cups cooked or canned black beans
- 1 avocado, sliced
- 1 to 1 1/2 cup enchilada sauce
- 1 to 1 1/2 cups cooked brown rice

- 6 flour tortillas, for burritos
- 6 handfuls green leaves

Directions:

1. Put the rice, black beans, and the enchilada sauce in a nonstick pan. Stir to combine and heat over very low heat. Check for salt, adding more as needed.

2. While the rice mixture is heating, heat the tortillas.

3. When the tortillas and the rice mixture are heated, spoon 1-2 tablespoons of the rice mixture on each tortilla. Top with avocado and the greens.

4. To fold the burritos, first fold the two sides towards the center and then starting from the bottom, roll them up, rolling until they are completely rolled up.

5. Wrap each with foil or parchment paper if you are taking them with you.

Notes: You can also add vegan cheese, tomato, vegan cream cheese, and cilantro to the filling.

Calories:	***476*** kcal
Total Carbohydrates:	***84*** g
Sugar:	***4.3*** g
Total Fat:	***9.1*** g
Protein:	***18.2*** g
Sodium:	***51*** mg

Healthy Hummus

Prep Time: **15** minutes

Cook Time: **0** minutes

Serves: **4**

Ingredients:

- 2 cans (15-ounces) garbanzo beans
- 1/2 teaspoon paprika
- 1/2 teaspoon cumin
- 1/2 cup lemon juice
- 2 cloves garlic, crushed
- 2 tablespoons chopped fresh parsley
- 4 teaspoons olive oil
- Salt, to taste

Directions:

1. Drain the beans, reserving 1/2 cup of the

liquid from the can and setting aside 1/4 cup of the garbanzo beans.

2. Put the rest of the garbanzo beans in a food processor or blender. Add the lemon juice and process or blend until the mixture is pureed.

3. Add the salt, cumin, paprika, parsley, garlic, and olive oil and process or blend again, adding the reserved bean liquid slowly until your preferred consistency is achieved. Transfer the pureed mixture into a bowl and stir in the reserved beans.

4. Refrigerate for 2 hours. Serve with some whole beans, parsley, veggies, bread, and chips or pita bread, or whatever dipping you desire.

Calories:	**826** kcal
Total Carbohydrates:	**130.5** g
Sugar:	**23.5** g
Total Fat:	**17.9** g
Protein:	**41.5** g
Sodium:	**98** mg

Fruity Quesadilla

Prep Time: **10** minutes

Cook Time: **4** minutes

Serves: **2-4**

Ingredients:

- 1 banana, thinly sliced
- 1 tablespoon maple syrup
- 1/2 cup thinly sliced apples
- 10-12 grapes
- 2 tablespoons coconut cream
- 2 whole-wheat flour tortillas
- 4 tablespoons peanut butter

Directions:

1. Spread the peanut butter on 1 tortilla. Layer the banana slices, grapes, and apple slices

on the peanut butter layer.

2. Combine the coconut cream and the maple syrup. Drizzle the mixture over the fruit and peanut butter layers.

3. Heat a skillet on medium-high heat and grease with cooking spray. Add the quesadilla and cook each side for about 2 minutes or until golden brown, carefully flipping the quesadilla.

4. Top with the other tortilla. Press firmly and then slice the quesadilla into quarters.

Calories:	**239** kcal
Total Carbohydrates:	**31.5** g
Sugar:	**13.7** g
Total Fat:	**11.3** g
Protein:	**6.6** g
Sodium:	**266** mg

Veggie Poppers to Adore

Prep Time: **10** minutes

Cook Time: **20** minutes

Serves: **6**

Ingredients:

- 1 can (4-ounces) green chilies, optional
- 1 teaspoon cumin
- 1/2 cup crushed toasted tortilla chips or red pepper flake, for garnish, optional
- 1/2 yellow or white onion, diced
- 10 jalapeños, halved, seeded, stems removed
- 2 cloves garlic, minced
- 2 tablespoons nutritional yeast
- 3/4 cup raw cashews, soaked in water for 4-6 hours or overnight, drained

- 3/4 cup veggie stock

- Olive oil

Directions:

1. Preheat the oven to 400F.

2. Slice the jalapenos into lengthwise halves, cut the tops off and then spray or brush with a bit of olive oil. With the cut side faced up, arrange them in a row.

3. If using crushed tortilla chips, spray them olive oil, and then bake them for about 7 to 10 minutes or until they are golden brown.

4. Grease a small-sized saucepan with olive oil and heat on medium heat. Add the garlic and onion, and sauté for about 5 minutes or until fragrant and just softened. Set aside.

5. Put the cashews, green chilies, vegetable stock, cumin, nutritional yeast, onion, and garlic into a blender and blend until smooth and creamy.

6. Pipe or spoon the cashew mixture into the jalapeno halves, filling them generously. Reserve leftover filling as a dip or for nachos.

7. Top the filling with the toasted, crushed tortilla chips if using. Bake in the oven for about 15 minutes or until the color of the filling has deepened and the jalapenos are soft.

8. Transfer the pan on the top rack. Broil for 1-2 minutes to intensify the flavor and color.

9. Serve right away, sprinkling with red pepper flakes if desired.

10. Notes: Store leftovers in covered containers ad keep refrigerated for a couple of days. When ready to serve, reheat in a preheated 350F oven or microwave until warmed through.

Calories:	**68** kcal
Total Carbohydrates:	**8** g
Sugar:	**3** g
Total Fat:	**3.7** g
Protein:	**2.2** g
Sodium:	**25** mg

Amazing Asparagus Quick Eat

Prep Time: **15-20** minutes

Cook Time: **20-25** minutes

Serves: **4**

Ingredients:

- 1 bunch asparagus
- 1 cup almond meal
- 1 teaspoon Himalayan pink salt
- 1 teaspoon maple syrup
- 1 teaspoon smoked paprika
- 1/2 teaspoon ground black pepper
- 2 tablespoons nutritional yeast, optional
- A drizzle of your preferred cooking oil

Directions:

1. Preheat the oven to 400F.

2. Wash the asparagus clean and slice into halves. Put into a deep bowl. Sprinkle with maple syrup, paprika, pepper, salt, and if using, with oil. Mix and toss to coat evenly.

3. Put the almond meal and if using, the nutritional yeast in a separate dish and mix to combine. Working with 1 piece at a time, put the asparagus in the almond meal and coat with the almond meal mixture.

4. Put the coated asparagus pieces on a parchment paper-lined baking sheet. Bake in the preheated oven to about 20 to 25 minutes or until golden brown.

5. Serve with your favorite dip.

Calories:	**182** kcal
Total Carbohydrates:	**12.8** g
Sugar:	**3.9** g
Total Fat:	**12.4** g
Protein:	**9.6** g
Sodium:	**766** mg

A Quick Apple Delight

Prep Time: *5* minutes

Cook Time: *0* minutes

Serves: *2*

Ingredients:

- 1 large granny smith apples, cored
- 1 tablespoon maple syrup
- 1/4 cup chunky peanut butter spread
- 2 tablespoons cranberries

Directions:

1. Put the peanut butter and the maple syrup in a small-sized bowl. Stir to combine and set aside.

2. Cut off 1/2-inch from the bottom and the top of the apples; discard the cut off parts.

3. Slice each apple into four round pieces.

Spread butter on 2 apple slices, sprinkle with the cranberries, and then top with the remaining apple slices. Enjoy!

Calories:	**260** kcal
Total Carbohydrates:	**28** g
Sugar:	**21** g
Total Fat:	**17** g
Protein:	**7** g
Sodium:	**125** mg

Break Time Crunch Rolls

Prep Time: **15** minutes

Cook Time: **45** minutes

Serves: **20** rolls

Ingredients:

- 1 medium-sized onion
- 1/2 teaspoon red chili powder
- 1/4 cup cilantro
- 1/4 teaspoon garam masala
- 1/4 teaspoon garlic powder
- 2 cups shredded cabbage
- 2 medium-sized carrots, spiralized
- 2 tablespoons tomato ketchup
- 2 teaspoons oil
- 20 sheets spring rolls

- 2-3 tablespoons soy sauce

- 3 tablespoons aquafaba, OR oil

- Salt, to taste

Directions:

1. Heat a pan over medium flame or heat. Add the oil and when the oil is hot, add the onion and sauté until transparent. Add the garlic powder and sauté.

2. Add the cabbage and carrots, and cook for 2 to 3 minutes or until half cooked. Add the garam masala and red chili powder, and sauté for 3 to 4 minutes.

3. Add the tomato ketchup, salt, soy sauce, and sauté for 2 minutes. Take the pan off the heat. Sprinkle with a couple of cilantro and let cool. DO NOT OVERWORK the veggies.

4. Take a sheet of spring roll. If they are not moist, sprinkle with a bit of water. Fill the roll with vegetables and roll, seal with cornstarch paste or water. Repeat with the

remaining filling and spring rolls.

5. Preheat the oven to 375F.

6. Put all the rolls on a greased baking sheet pan. Lightly brush the rolls with aquafaba or oil.

7. Bake in the preheated oven for about 20 to 25 minutes or until golden and crispy.

Calories:	**151** kcal
Total Carbohydrates:	**14.1** g
Sugar:	**2.8** g
Total Fat:	**9.5** g
Protein:	**2.9** g
Sodium:	**278** mg

Creative Cookies

Prep Time: *10* minutes

Cook Time: *8-15* minutes

Serves: *24* cookies

Ingredients:

- 3 very ripe bananas (around 1 1/2 cups mashed or pureed until smooth)
- 1/2 cup cocoa powder
- 1/2 cup unsweetened natural creamy peanut butter, OR almond butter
- Small handful of coarse sea salt, for garnish

Directions:

1. Preheat the oven to 350F.
2. Put the bananas, cocoa powder, and peanut butter in a large-sized mixing bowl and combine using a fork until the mixture is

uniform and smooth. Alternatively, you can process in a food processor for about 30 to 60 seconds.

3. By heaping tablespoons, scoop the dough into a parchment paper lined or greased cookie sheet, placing the dough 1 inch apart.

4. Sprinkle the cookie tops with a pinch of salt. Bake in the preheated oven for about 8 to 15 minutes or until the cookies lose their sheen.

5. When the cookies are baked, let them cool on the cookie sheet for about 3 to 5 minutes. Transfer onto a wire rack and let cool completely.

Notes: If the batter is too thin, you can add more cocoa powder to absorb the moisture and/or bake longer. If your peanut butter is too tough, you can microwave it for 15 to 20 seconds until smooth and easier to work with. Make sure you mix the peanut butter thoroughly in the mixture. If you don't want to garnish the cookies with salt, add 1 pinch salt to the batter.

Calories:	*42* kcal
Total Carbohydrates:	*4.1* g
Sugar:	*1.5* g
Total Fat:	*2.9* g
Protein:	*1.4* g
Sodium:	*0* mg

Great Guacamole

Prep Time: **10** minutes

Cook Time: **0** minutes

Serves: **6-8**

Ingredients:

- 3 medium-sized ripe avocados
- 1-2 pinches coarse salt
- 1/4 cup red onion, finely chopped
- 1/4 cup cilantro leaves, chopped
- 1/2 jalapeño pepper, minced, less or more to taste
- 1 lime, juice only

Directions:

1. Slice the avocado into halves and remove the pit.

2. Spoon the avocado meat into a mixing bowl.

3. Add the salt, cilantro, jalapeno, and onion, and mix to combine.

4. Add the lime juice and gently stir so that you don't crush the ingredients aggressively.

Calories:	**150** kcal
Total Carbohydrates:	**10** g
Sugar:	**1** g
Total Fat:	**13** g
Protein:	**2** g
Sodium:	**5** mg

Bright Banana Mash

Prep Time: *5* minutes

Cook Time: *30* minutes

Serves: *1*

Ingredients:

- 1 very ripe banana, mashed
- 1/2 teaspoon pure vanilla extract
- 1/4 cup almond milk, OR your preferred milk
- 1/4 cup dry quinoa
- 1/4 teaspoon cinnamon
- 2 tablespoons walnuts

Directions:

1. Cook the quinoa following the package directions.

2. When the quinoa is cooked, reduce the heat to low. Stir in the mashed banana, milk, cinnamon, and vanilla. As desired, mix the walnuts into the quinoa mixture or serve them topped on the mixture.

3. Serve while still warm. Enjoy!

Notes: Add more milk as need to achieve desired texture.

Calories:	*503* kcal
Total Carbohydrates:	*59.8* g
Sugar:	*16.9* g
Total Fat:	*26.5* g
Protein:	*12.4* g
Sodium:	*13* mg

Chapter 8: Divine Desserts

There's always room for these sweet treats. These plant-based will excite your taste buds, but are good for your health, too.

Carrot Cake to Go

Prep Time: *1* hour

Cook Time: *0* minutes

Serves: ***8-10***

Ingredients:

For the cashew frosting:

- 1/3 cup pure maple syrup
- 1-2 tablespoons fresh squeezed lemon juice
- 2 cups cashews, soaked in water for a couple of hours or overnight

- 2 tablespoons liquid coconut oil
- Water, as needed

For the cake:

- 1 1/2 cups oat flour, OR buckwheat flour
- 1 cup dates, pitted
- 1 cup dried pineapple
- 1/2 cup unsweetened dried coconut
- 1/2 teaspoon ground cinnamon
- 2 large carrots, peeled

Directions:

For the cashew frosting:

1. Put all of the ingredients into a high-powered blender and blend until the mixtures smooth, adding as little water as possible. Taste and add more maple syrup as desired. Transfer to a bowl. Set aside.

For the cake:

1. Slice the carrots into small-sized chunks.

2. Put the carrot chunks into a food processor. Add the rest of the ingredients and pulse until the ingredients into very small pieces that stick together.

To assemble:

1. Press 1/2 of the cake mixture into the bottom of an adjustable 6-inch spring-form pan, spreading into an even layer. Spread about 1/3 of the frosting on the cake mixture. Press the remaining 1/2 cake mixture on top of the frosting layer.

2. At this point you can refrigerate the cake overnight before frosting or frost right away.

3. Remove the cake from the pan and cover with the remaining frosting, garnishing the cake with whatever you want.

Calories: *438* kcal

Total Carbohydrates: *53.7* g

Sugar: **25.5** g

Total Fat: **23.5** g

Protein: **8.9** g

Sodium: **21** mg

Cool Strawberry Cupcakes

Prep Time: **15** minutes

Cook Time: **45** minutes

Serves: **12-16** cupcakes or **2** pieces 9-inch cakes

Ingredients:

- 8 ounces strawberries, fresh or frozen, crushed or pureed
- 3/4-1 cup sugar
- 1/2 cup canola oil
- 1 teaspoon vanilla extract
- 1 teaspoon baking soda
- 1 tablespoon white distilled vinegar
- 1 3/4 cups unbleached all-purpose flour

Directions:

1. Preheat the oven to 350F for 15 minutes.

2. Line or grease 12-16 muffin tin cups or grease a 9-inch loaf pan. Set aside.

3. Put the flour, sugar, and baking soda in a large-sized bowl and mix until combined.

4. In a different bowl, put the vanilla, vinegar, and oil, and stir to mix. Add the strawberry and stir to incorporate.

5. Create a well in the center of the flour mixture. Add the vanilla mixture into the well and stir to combine until just mixed. DO NOT OVERSTIR.

6. Pour the batter into the prepared muffin tin cups or the loaf pan.

7. Bake in the preheated oven for about 22-30 minutes for muffins and 40 minutes-1 hour for a loaf or until a toothpick comes out clean when inserted in the center of the muffins or the loaf.

8. When cooked, remove from the oven and put on a wire rack and let cool.

9. When completely cool, frost the cupcakes and then top each with 1 whole piece strawberry.

Calories:	**160** kcal
Total Carbohydrates:	**21** g
Sugar:	**15** g
Total Fat:	**8** g
Protein:	**<1** g
Sodium:	**90** mg

Must-Have Gingerbread

Prep Time: **25** minutes

Cook Time: **35** minutes

Serves: **12**

Ingredients:

- 1 cup unsweetened applesauce
- 1 teaspoon baking powder
- 1 teaspoon baking soda
- 1 teaspoon ground cinnamon
- 1/2 cup unsulfured molasses
- 1/3 cup coconut oil
- 1/3 cup potato starch, NOT FLOUR
- 1/4 teaspoon ground cloves
- 1/4 teaspoon salt
- 2 tablespoons ground flax seeds

- 2 teaspoons ground ginger

- 2/3 cup coconut palm sugar

- 5/6 cup millet flour

- 5/6 cup teff flour

- 6 tablespoons warm water

Directions:

1. Preheat the oven to 350F. Grease a square 8-inch pan or line it with parchment paper.

2. Put the ground flax seeds into a small-sized bowl. Add the water and stir until the mixture is creamy and thick. Set aside and let stand for at least 10 minutes.

3. Except for the coconut palm sugar, sift all the dry ingredients into a large-sized mixing bowl.

4. In a different mixing bowl, put the flax mixture, applesauce, coconut oil, molasses, and coconut palm sugar, and whisk until well combined. Add the wet mixture to the

bowl with the dry ingredients. Stir until blended.

5. Pour the batter into the pan and then bake for about 35 minutes or until set and a toothpick inserted in the center comes out clean.

6. Let the gingerbread cool in the pan on a wire rack.

7. When the bread is cool enough to handle, turn the pan and remove the bread from the pan.

8. Best eaten on the same day, but you can refrigerate any leftovers.

Calories:	***210*** kcal
Total Carbohydrates:	***35*** g
Sugar:	***18*** g
Total Fat:	***9*** g
Protein:	***3*** g
Sodium:	***210*** mg

Fabulous Fruit Squares

Prep Time: **15** minutes

Cook Time: **40** minutes

Serves: **16** bars

Ingredients:

For the topping and crust:

- 1 1/2 cups rolled oats
- 1 tablespoon lemon zest
- 1/2 cup raw sugar, OR brown sugar
- 2/3 cup coconut oil, at room temperature
- 1/4 teaspoon baking powder
- 1/4 teaspoon salt
- 3/4 cup ivory whole-wheat flour, OR all-purpose flour

For the filling:

- 1/2 teaspoon vanilla extract

- 2 1/2 cups fresh blueberries, DO NOT USE FROZEN

- 7 tablespoons raspberry jam, OR your preferred berry jam

- Pinch salt

Directions:

1. Preheat the oven to 375F.

2. Line a square 8-inch baking pan with parchment paper.

3. Put the oats, salt, baking powder, lemon zest, sugar, and flour into a large-sized bow, and mix to combine well.

4. Add the coconut oil. With clean hands, mix until the mixture is a dough. It should stick together and not very crumbly.

5. Gently press less than 2/3 of the dough on the bottom of the prepared baking pan.

6. Bake in the preheated oven for about 10 to13 minutes or until the edges begin to brown.

7. While the crust is baking, prepare the filling. Put the salt, vanilla extract, jam, and berries into a medium-sized bowl and mix to combine.

8. Spoon filling into the freshly baked crust and sprinkle the remaining oat mixture on top of the filling.

9. Bake for 22 to 27 minutes more or until the filling is bubbly and the top is lightly browned.

10. Remove from the oven and let cool completely. Transfer into the refrigerator and chill for at least 2 hours. Slice into 16 bars. Enjoy!

11. Refrigerate any leftovers for up to 4 days or freeze for longer storage.

Notes: If the coconut oil is melted or liquid at

room temperature, mix the topping and crust ingredients. Refrigerate for about 10 to 20 minutes or until the mixture is frim enough to press on the bottom of the pan.

Calories:	**188** kcal
Total Carbohydrates:	**25** g
Sugar:	**12.6** g
Total Fat:	**9.7** g
Protein:	**1.8** g
Sodium:	**47** mg

Colorful Parfait

Prep Time: **15** minutes

Cook Time: **0** minutes

Serves: **2**

Ingredients:

For the cashew cream:

- 1 cup raw unsalted cashews, soaked in water for 2 hours
- 1 teaspoon natural vanilla extract, plus more as needed
- 1/2 cup filtered water, plus more as needed
- 2 tablespoons pure maple syrup, plus more as needed
- Pinch Celtic sea salt

For the nut and seed mix:

- 1/4 cup shredded coconut, unsweetened

dried

- 1/4 cup shelled hemp seeds
- 1/4 cup raw sunflower seeds
- 1/4 cup raw pumpkin seeds
- 1 cup raw walnuts
- 1 cup raw almonds

For the berries:

- 1 cup fresh raspberries
- 1 cup fresh blueberries

Directions:

For the cashew cream:

1. Drain the cashews, discarding the soaking water. Put the cashews in a high-powered blender. Add the rest of the ingredients and blend for about 30-60 seconds or until creamy and smooth. Taste and add more vanilla, sweetener, and water to suit your taste.

2. Transfer into a sealed container, refrigerate, and chill for a couple of hours to thicken.

For the nut and seed mix:

1. Put all of the ingredients into a food processor and pulse a couple of times until the nuts are chopped and chunky.

To assemble:

1. Prepare 2 short, wide glasses. Put 1/2 cup blueberries in each glass. Spoon 1/4 cup of the nut-seed mixture, 1/2 of the cashew cream, 1/4 cup of the nut-seed mixture into each glass and then finish with 1/2 cup raspberries for each glass.

2. Serve right away.

Calories: *1359* kcal

Total Carbohydrates: *76* g

Sugar: *29.2* g

Total Fat: *108.2* g

Protein: *43.3* g

Sodium: *101* mg

Precious Pudding

Prep Time: *5* minutes

Cook Time: *0* minutes

Serves: *2*

Ingredients:

- 1 avocado
- 1 banana
- 1 teaspoon vanilla extract, optional
- 1/2 cup maple syrup
- 1/2 cup unsweetened cocoa powder
- 1/4 cup rice milk

For topping:

- Caramel syrup
- Coconut whipped cream

Directions:

1. Put all of the ingredients into a blender or a food processor and blend or process until the mixture is smooth.

2. Divide the pudding between 2 serving glasses.

3. Chill for at least 2 hours or up to overnight, or serve right away.

4. Top with coconut whipped cream and drizzle with caramel syrup.

Calories: **662** kcal

Total Carbohydrates: **106.2** g

Sugar: **70.2** g

Total Fat: **30.3** g

Protein: **7.5** g

Sodium: **44** mg

Mouthwatering Chocolate Gelato

Prep Time: *5* minutes

Cook Time: *0* minutes

Serves: *2-3*

Ingredients:

- 1 cup dates, pitted, soaked in water or the coconut water from the coconut milk can until very soft

- 1 cup frozen banana pieces

- 1 cup refrigerated coconut cream, from 1 can of regular coconut milk

- 1/4 teaspoon sea salt

- 1/4-1/2 teaspoon vanilla bean powder, OR seeds from 1 vanilla bean or 1/2 teaspoon vanilla extract, optional

- 3 tablespoons cocoa powder

Directions:

1. Put all of the ingredients into a high-powered blender and blend until very smooth.

2. Transfer the mixture into a container and freeze for about 2-3 hours for gelato-like texture or 4 to 5 hours for a firmer texture.

3. Notes: Refrigerate the coconut milk overnight or a couple of days. The coconut cream will rise to the top and will be easy to scoop out.

Calories:	**615** kcal
Total Carbohydrates:	**95.1** g
Sugar:	**69.8** g
Total Fat:	**30.3** g
Protein:	**7.2 g**
Sodium:	**256** mg

Datable Dates

Prep Time: *1* hour, *25* minutes

Cook Time: *0* minutes

Serves: *16* bars

Ingredients:

For the crust:

- 10 Medjool dates, pitted, roughly chopped
- 1/4 cup coconut oil, melted
- 1/2 teaspoon kosher salt
- 1 1/2 cups whole pieces raw almonds
- 1 1/2 cups regular oats

For the filling:

- 1/2 cup water
- 25 Medjool dates, pitted, roughly chopped, about 2 1/2 cups

Directions:

1. Line a square 8-inch pan with 2 pieces of parchment paper, placing them opposite ways.

2. Put the oats, salt, and almond in a food processor and process until it forms into a fine crumble.

3. Add the dates and process until crumbly.

4. Add the coconut oil and process until the mixture is sticky, adding a bit more oil as needed to achieve the right consistency.

5. Transfer into a bowl, setting aside 3/4 cup of the mixture. Press the rest of the oat mixture into a firm and very firm layer into the pan.

6. Put the dates and water in the food processor and process until the texture is pasty, stopping and scraping the sides down as needed. Add a bit more water as needed to achieve the right consistency.

7. Scoop the date mixture into the crust and spread gently with the back of a wet spatula into an even layer.

8. Sprinkle the reserved 3/4 cup reserved oat mixture on top of the date filling, pressing gently with your fingers.

9. Refrigerate for at least 1 hour, preferably overnight, until set and firm.

10. Slice into squares and serve. Store leftovers in the refrigerator or freezer.

Calories:	***408*** kcal
Total Carbohydrates:	***64.3*** g
Sugar:	***43.2*** g
Total Fat:	***17*** g
Protein:	***7.4 g***
Sodium:	***150*** mg

Pretty Pumpkin Pie

Prep Time: **6** hours, **10** minutes

Cook Time: **35** minutes

Serves: **4-6**

Ingredients:

- 1 can (15-ounces) pumpkin puree
- 1 tablespoon ground flax
- 1 teaspoon pumpkin pie spice
- 1/2 teaspoon salt
- 1/3 cup flour
- 1/3 cup PLUS 2 tablespoons brown sugar
- 2 1/2 teaspoons pure vanilla extract
- 2 tablespoons oil, OR omit and increase milk to 1 cup
- 2 teaspoons baking powder

- 2 teaspoons cinnamon

- 3/4 cup PLUS 2 tablespoons milk

Directions:

1. Preheat the oven to 400F.

2. Grease a 10-inch round pie pan with oil.

3. Put the pumpkin pie spice, cinnamon, salt, baking powder, flour, 1/3 cup brown sugar, and pumpkin puree in a large-sized bowl and stir to combine well.

4. In another bowl, combine the flax with the all the wet ingredients, whisking to combine well.

5. Pour the wet ingredients into the dry ingredients, and stir to combine well.

6. Pour the batter into the prepared pan and bake in the oven for 35 minutes.

7. The pie will be gooey after the cooking time, which is perfectly alright. Let cool completely and then refrigerate uncovered

for at least 6 hours or until completely set.

8. Slice and serve.

Calories:	**246** kcal
Total Carbohydrates:	**38.7** g
Sugar:	**22.4** g
Total Fat:	**8.9** g
Protein:	**4.5** g
Sodium:	**329** mg

Berry Tempting Tarts

Prep Time: **10** minutes

Cook Time: **2** minutes

Serves: **4-6**

Ingredients:

For the crust:

- 1 1/2 cups almond flour
- 1 tablespoon pure maple syrup
- 1/4 cup coconut oil, melted
- 1/4 cup unsweetened cocoa powder
- Pinch kosher salt

For the filling:

- 6 ounces bittersweet chocolate, finely chopped
- 2 cups fresh raspberries

- 1/4 cup 100% fruit raspberry preserves

- 1/2 cup canned full-fat coconut milk

Directions:

1. Lightly grease a 9-inch tart pan with a removable bottom with the coconut oil.

2. Put all of the crust ingredients in a bowl and stir to combine well. Press into the greased tart pan into an even layer. Set aside.

3. Put the chocolate in a large-sized bowl.

4. Pour the coconut milk into a small-sized saucepan and bring to just a boil.

5. Pour the hot coconut milk over the chopped chocolate. Let stand for 1 minute and stir until creamy and smooth.

6. Stir in the raspberry preserves and pour the filling into the prepared crust. Garnish the top with the raspberries.

7. Refrigerate the tart for at least 1 to 2 hours or until completely cool and set.

8. Slice and serve.

Notes: Put any leftover in airtight containers and store in the refrigerator.

Calories:	***758 kcal***
Total Carbohydrates:	***62.6*** g
Sugar:	***39.4*** g
Total Fat:	***54.4*** g
Protein:	***14.6*** g
Sodium:	***88*** mg

Chapter 9: The 14-Day Getting Started Meal Plan

There is no pressure to create a fancy and complicated menu on the plant-based diet. A complicated dish and meal plan will only intimidate and dishearten you on your journey to a healthy lifestyle. Your success in transitioning to this healthy eating habit is to stick to the basics and to keep things simple. There are hundreds of simple, straightforward recipes that will inspire and excite your taste buds. You can start with the ones featured in this book.

Understand Planning is Vital

It is important to understand that when you start reducing or eliminating animal-based foods to a plant-based diet, it will be difficult to consume the adequate amounts of nutrients that you usually take in your body, including dietary protein, as well as a wide range of minerals and vitamins.

According to the American Dietetic Association, careful planning is needed to make sure that you avoid the common nutrient deficiencies you may experience. A well-planned menu is appropriate for all individuals during all stages of their life cycle, including infancy, childhood, adolescence, even for athletes, as well as pregnant and lactating women.

You need to make sure you get enough of the following nutrients:

- **Protein** – Most people need to get 1/3 of their daily calorie needs from protein. If you are training, active, or if you are an athlete, you need to consume at least 0.75-0.80 grams of protein per pound of your body weight as a base. Quinoa, seeds, nuts, legumes, and beans are excellent sources of dietary protein.

- **Vitamin B 12** – Aim for about 3 to 5 microgram daily from plant-based food or take 10-100 microgram supplement daily. You can get vitamin B 12 from nutritional yeast and fortified plant-based products.

- **Vitamin D** – Aim for 1000-4000 IU during winter months and days that you do not get any sunshine. Sunlight is the best source of vitamin D. You can supplement with D2, which are animal free vitamin D supplements.

- **Calcium** – Aim for about 1000 milligrams daily. You can get it from fortified nondairy milk, calcium-set tofu, seeds, nuts, beans, and dark leafy greens.

- **Iodine** - Aim for around 1000 milligrams daily. You can get iodine from iodized salt, green leafy vegetables, asparagus, sea vegetables, and kelp.

- **Omega-3 fatty acids** – Consume at least 2 grams daily of alpha-linolenic acid (ALA), a type of omega-3 fatty acid found in plants. If possible, add eicosapentaenoic acid (EPA) and docosahexaenoic acid (DHA) from algae supplements and not from fish oil. You can get plant-based omega-3 fatty acid from green leafy vegetables, walnuts, hemp, flax, and algae supplements.

The key to a successful plant-based diet, or any diet, is to make sure you consume a well-balanced meal. And planning ahead of time ensures that you start your new healthy lifestyle on the right track.

2 Weeks of Plant-Based Dishes

To start your plant-based diet journey, keep things simple. Reduce the amount of ingredients for each recipe to serve 2 people. This plan involves consuming today's meal and then saving the leftovers as your meal for the day after tomorrow. However, you can also cook each dish following the number of servings indicated and share the extra with friends and family. You might even inspire them to go on a healthy journey together with you. Dieting with a friend is always better.

Week 1

Day 1

Breakfast: Oats to Love

Lunch: The Most Desirable Chili Bowl

Snack: Healthy Hummus with whole beans, parsley, veggies, bread, and chips or pita bread, or whatever dipping you desire

Dinner: A Tempeh Treat

Dessert: Mouthwatering Chocolate Gelato

Day 2

Breakfast: Granola Energizer

Lunch: Plant Based Meatloaf

Snack: Burrito Bites

Dinner: Vietnamese Noodles for the Soul

Dessert: Carrot Cake to Go

Day 3

Leftovers from Day 1

Breakfast: Oats to Love

Lunch: The Most Desirable Chili Bowl

Snack: Healthy Hummus with whole beans, parsley, veggies, bread, and chips or pita bread, or whatever dipping you desire OR leftovers

Dinner: A Tempeh Treat

Dessert: Mouthwatering Chocolate Gelato

Day 4

Leftovers from Day 2

Breakfast: Granola Energizer

Lunch: Plant Based Meatloaf

Snack: Burrito Bites

Dinner: Vietnamese Noodles for the Soul

Dessert: Carrot Cake to Go

Day 5

Breakfast: The Pancake Solution

Lunch: Curried Potatoes in Thai Style

Snack: Veggie Poppers to Adore

Dinner: Effortlessly Made Pizza

Dessert: Berry Tempting Tarts

Day 6

Breakfast: The Energy Porridge

Lunch: Perfect Pineapple Fried Rice

Snack: Break Time Crunch Rolls

Dinner: Plant-Based Casserole

Dessert: Precious Pudding

Day 7

Leftovers from Day 5

Breakfast: The Pancake Solution

Lunch: Curried Potatoes in Thai Style, OR leftovers

Snack: Veggie Poppers to Adore

Dinner: Effortlessly Made Pizza

Dessert: Berry Tempting Tarts

Week 2

Day 1

Leftovers from Week 1 Day 6

Breakfast: The Energy Porridge

Lunch: Perfect Pineapple Fried Rice, OR leftovers

Snack: Break Time Crunch Rolls

Dinner: Plant-Based Casserole

Dessert: Precious Pudding

Day 2

Breakfast: Start the Day with Salad

Lunch: A Valuable Vegetable Quiche

Snack: Bright Banana Mash

Dinner: A Surprising Stew

Dessert: Datable Dates

Day 3

Breakfast: Rich Rice Pudding

Lunch: A Vegetable Wrap Wonder

Snack: Creative Cookies

Dinner: Oh My! Bulgur Pilaf

Dessert: Colorful Parfait

Day 4

Leftovers from Day 2

Breakfast: Start the Day with Salad

Lunch: A Valuable Vegetable Quiche

Snack: Bright Banana Mash

Dinner: A Surprising Stew

Dessert: Datable Dates

Day 5

Leftovers from Day 3

Breakfast: Rich Rice Pudding

Lunch: A Vegetable Wrap Wonder

Snack: Creative Cookies

Dinner: Oh My! Bulgur Pilaf

Dessert: Colorful Parfait

Day 6

Breakfast: Merry to Eat Muffins

Lunch: Tasty Tofu

Snack: Break Time Crunch Rolls

Dinner: A Nutritious Pasta Plate

Dessert: Fabulous Fruit Squares

Day 7

Breakfast: A Delightful Chickpea Omelet Plate

Lunch: A Triple-B Burger

Snack: A Quick Apple Delight

Dinner: Sweet Potatoes and Kale from Africa

Dessert: Cool Strawberry Cupcakes

Establish Success with Your Health Goals

Transitioning to a plant-based diet is one of the most beneficial things you can do for yourself, but is it as simple as it sounds? Like many other diets, changing your diet can look pretty intimidating, especially when you switch into a healthy eating habit from being an omnivore your entire life. Most of us grew up where our regular meals included beef, pork, chicken, eggs, dairy, and other animal-based food at every single meal. They key to success is planning your transition. Here are essential and practical tips to help you transition from an animal-based diet to a plant-based one.

- **Educate Yourself**

  Your best chance to succeed in any diet is to educate yourself and learn everything you need to know about this healthy eating habit. Don't do it because it is the fad. Do it because you see all the health benefits you will get from eating whole foods. Learn how other people who have successfully transitioned. Learning all you can about the advantages of more fruits and vegetables will motivate you and knowing how others successfully changed their diet and will give you confidence in your transition. The key to transitioning to a new eating plan is to be excited about it.

- **Focus on Crowding Out, Not Cutting Out**

  It is all about perspective. If you focus on not buying dairy, eggs, and meat when you are at the grocery store, you will feel deprived and defeated. However, if your mindset is all about filling your kitchen with healthy plant-based food, such as berries, almonds, coconut milk, flax, mushrooms, tomatoes, bananas, sweet potatoes, spinach, kale, and quinoa, then it will feel like you are shopping food for a fancy menu.

  Crowd out animal-based foods with legumes, seeds, nuts, whole grains, vegetables, fruits, and nondairy milk, avoiding vegan meat replacement as much as you can. Remember that this diet focuses on meals rich in whole foods.

- **Find Creative Plant-Based Recipes to Inspire You**

When you first hear about a plant-based diet, you will often think of steamed broccoli and salad. However, when you research for plant-based recipes, you will find many simple and straightforward, yet very creative and incredibly tasty plant-based meals. The 50 fabulous recipes in this book will motivate and inspire you with zeal and zest as you change to a healthy lifestyle.

- **Focus on the Basics**

Eating a meal rich in whole foods does not have to be complicated and hard. Start with basic, simple, and easy recipes for your first batch of meals. For example, you can start your day with Oats to Love, a simple dish with Chia seeds, almond milk, blueberries, and agave nectar to sweeten. For lunch, recipes that you can refrigerate and grab to go like "The Most Desirable Chili Bowl", salads, and soups are excellent choices. Sliced vegetables and fruits with raw walnuts and almonds are great snacks. Your dinner can be "A Tempeh Treat", a simple dish with microgreens and healthy avocado. You can treat yourself to Mouthwatering Chocolate Gelato after your meal.

Remember, it does not have to be fancy. The basic ingredients can be as tasty. When in doubt, you can always make a delicious smoothie. They can fill the gaps and keep things interesting and creative, not to mention scrumptious.

- **Take it One Step at a Time**

You do not have to overwhelm yourself, create a sophisticated meal plan, or prepare complicated dishes when you are transitioning to a plant-based diet. Take it meal after meal, and then day by day. There is no need to be intimidated or stressed about going on this healthy food plan. You will have more success if you stick to more straightforward dishes and meals.

- **Stick to Whole Foods**

    It's easy to go plant-based and by processed plant-based foods, but that is not the best way to change into a healthy diet. Always choose whole foods. Avoid refined carbohydrates, processed meat substitutes, and other highly processed products. Moreover, do not consume junk food just because they are labeled vegan or vegetarian.

- **Consume a Wide Variety of Plant-Based Food**

    To keep your diet balanced and provide you with all the nutrients you need, consume a wide variety of plant-based foods, not just a handful.

    Now that you are beginning your journey to a healthier eating habit, success is enviable when you keep all these important elements in mind.

Final Words

Thank you again for purchasing this book! I really hope this book is able to help you.

The next step is for you to **join our email newsletter** to receive updates on any upcoming new book releases or promotions. You can sign-up for free and as a bonus, you will also receive our "*7 Fitness Mistakes You Don't Know You're Making*" book! This bonus book breaks down many of the most common fitness mistakes and will demystify many of the complexities and science of getting into shape. Having all this fitness knowledge and science organized into an actionable step-by-step book will help you get started in the right direction in your fitness journey! To join our free email newsletter and grab your free book, please visit the link and signup: www.hmwpublishing.com/gift

Finally, if you enjoyed this book, then I would like to ask you for a favor, would you be kind enough to leave a review for this book? It would be greatly appreciated!

Thank you and good luck in your journey!

About the Co-Author

My name is George Kaplo; I'm a certified personal trainer from Montreal, Canada. I'll start off by saying I'm not the biggest guy you will ever meet and this has never really been my goal. In fact, I started working out to overcome my biggest insecurity when I was younger, which was my self-confidence. This was due to my height measuring only 5 foot 5 inches (168cm), it pushed me down to attempt anything I ever wanted to achieve in life. You may be going through some challenges right now, or you may simply want to get fit, and I can certainly relate.

For me personally, I was always kind of interested

in the health & fitness world and wanted to gain some muscle due to the numerous bullying in my teenage years about my height and my overweight body. I figured I couldn't do anything about my height, but I sure can do something about how my body looked like. This was the beginning of my transformation journey. I had no idea where to start, but I just got started. I felt worried and afraid at times that other people would make fun of me for doing the exercises the wrong way. I always wished I had a friend that was next to me who was knowledgeable enough to help me get started and "show me the ropes."

After a lot of work, studying and countless trial and errors. Some people began to notice how I was getting more fit and how I was starting to form a keen interest in the topic. This led many friends and new faces to come to me and ask me for fitness advice. At first, it seemed odd when people asked me to help them get in shape. But what kept me going is when they started to see changes in their own body and told me it's the first time that they saw real results! From there, more people kept coming to me, and it made me realize after so much reading and studying in this field that it did help me but it also allowed me to help others. I'm now a fully certified personal trainer and have trained numerous clients to date who have achieved amazing results.

Today, my brother Alex Kaplo (also a Certified Personal Trainer) and I own & operate this publishing venture, where we bring passionate and expert authors to write about health and fitness topics. We also run an online fitness website "HelpMeWorkout.com" and I would love to connect with by inviting you to visit the website on the following page and signing up to our e-mail newsletter (you will even get a free book).

Last but not least, if you are in the position I was once in and you want some guidance, don't hesitate and ask... I'll be there to help you out!

Your friend and coach,

George Kaplo

Certified Personal Trainer

Get another book for Free

I want to thank you for purchasing this book and offer you another book (just as long and valuable as this book), "Health & Fitness Mistakes You Don't Know You're Making", completely free.

Visit the link below to signup and receive it:

www.hmwpublishing.com/gift

In this book, I will break down the most common health & fitness mistakes, you are probably committing right now, and I will reveal how you can easily get in the best shape of your life!

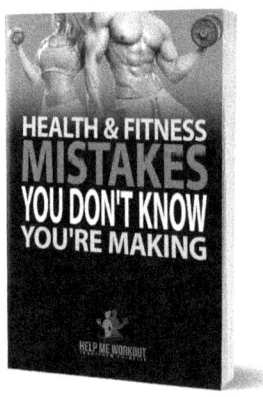

In addition to this valuable gift, you will also have an opportunity to get our new books for free, enter giveaways, and receive other valuable emails from me. Again, visit the link to sign up:

www.hmwpublishing.com/gift

Copyright 2017 by HMW Publishing - All Rights Reserved.

This document by HMW Publishing owned by the A&G Direct Inc company, is geared towards providing exact and reliable information in regards to the topic and issue covered. The publication is sold with the idea that the publisher is not required to render accounting, officially permitted, or otherwise, qualified services. If advice is necessary, legal or professional, a practiced individual in the profession should be ordered.

From a Declaration of Principles which was accepted and approved equally by a Committee of the American Bar Association and a Committee of Publishers and Associations.

In no way is it legal to reproduce, duplicate, or transmit any part of this document in either electronic means or in printed format. Recording of this publication is strictly prohibited, and any storage of this document is not allowed unless with written permission from the publisher. All rights reserved.

The information provided herein is stated to be truthful and consistent, in that any liability, in terms of inattention or otherwise, by any usage or abuse of any policies, processes, or directions contained within is the solitary and utter responsibility of the recipient reader. Under no circumstances will any legal responsibility or blame be held against the publisher for any reparation, damages, or monetary loss due to the information herein, either directly or indirectly.

The information herein is offered for informational purposes solely, and is universal as so. The presentation of the information is without contract or any type of guarantee assurance.

The trademarks that are used are without any consent, and the publication of the trademark is without permission or backing by the trademark owner. All trademarks and brands within this book are for clarifying purposes only and are the owned by the owners themselves, not affiliated with this document.

For more great books visit:

HMWPublishing.com

www.ingramcontent.com/pod-product-compliance
Lightning Source LLC
Chambersburg PA
CBHW071802080526
44589CB00012B/647